CANADIAN MEDICAL LIVES

WILLIAM BOYD
Silver Tongue and Golden Pen

Ian Carr

Series Editor: T.P. Morley

Associated Medical Services, Inc.
&
Fitzhenry & Whiteside
1993

Copyright © Associated Medical Services Incorporated/The Hannah Institute for the History of Medicine, 1993

Fitzhenry & Whiteside
195 Allstate Parkway
Markham, Ontario L3R 4T8

All rights reserved. No part of this publication may be reproduced, stored in a retrieval system, or transmitted in any form or by any means, electronic, mechanical, photocopying, recording, or otherwise, except brief passages for purposes of review, without the prior permission of Fitzhenry & Whiteside.

Jacket design: Anne Roosman
Copy Editor: Frank English
Printing and Binding: Gagné Printing Ltd., Louiseville, Quebec, Canada

Fitzhenry & Whiteside wishes to acknowledge the generous assistance and ongoing support of **The Book Publishing Industry Development Programme** of the **Department of Communications, The Canada Council,** and **The Ontario Arts Council.**

Care has been taken to trace the ownership of copyright material used in the text, including the illustrations. The author and publisher welcome any information enabling them to rectify any reference or credit in subsequent editions.

Canadian Cataloguing in Publication Data

Carr, Ian, 1932-
  William Boyd

(Canadian medical lives : no. 15)
Includes bibliographical references and index.
ISBN 1-55041-137-3

1. Boyd, William, 1885-1979. 2. Pathologists—Canada—Biography. I. Hannah Institute for the History of Medicine. II. Title. III. Series.

RB17.B6C3 1993   616.07'092   C93-094419-4

CANADIAN MEDICAL LIVES SERIES

The story of the Hannah Institute for the History of Medicine has been told by John B. Neilson and G.R. Paterson in *Associated Medical Services Incorporated: A History* (1987). Dr. Donald R. Wilson, President of AMS, and the Board of Directors decided that the Institute should produce this series of biographies as one of its undertakings.

The first ten biographies have now been published and can be obtained through the retail book trade or from Dundurn Press Ltd., 2181 Queen Street East, Suite 301, Toronto, Canada, M4E 1E5, and Dundurn Distribution, 73 Lime Walk, Headington, Oxford, England, OX3 7AD. The second group, of which this is the first volume, can also be obtained through retail book stores or from the publisher, Fitzhenry and Whiteside.

William Boyd, trainee psychiatrist turned self-taught pathologist, was venerated by students who attended his lectures and no less by those around the world who read his textbooks. Professor Ian Carr, never having sat at Boyd's feet when a medical student, is able to preserve some objectivity; but as a pathologist and, like Boyd, a Scot, he enters faithfully into the life of his subject.

Future volumes include *J.C.Boileau Grant* (C.L.N. Robinson), *R.M. Bucke* (Peter Rechnitzer), *William Henry Drummond* (J.B. Lyons) and *William Beaumont* (Julian Smith).

There is no shortage of meritorious subjects. Willing and capable authors are harder to acquire. The Institute is therefore deeply grateful to authors who have committed their time and skill to the series.

T.P. Morley
Series Editor
1993

CANADIAN MEDICAL LIVES SERIES

Duncan Graham by Robert B. Kerr and Douglas Waugh

Bill Mustard by Marilyn Dunlop

Joe Doupe by Terence Moore

Emily Stowe by Mary Beacock Fryer

Clarence Hincks by Charles G. Roland

Francis A.C. Scringer, V.C., by Suzanne Kingsmill

Earle P. Scarlett by F.W. Musselwhite

R.G. Ferguson by Stuart Houston

Harold Griffith by Richard Bodman and Deirdre Gillies

Maude Abbott by Douglas Waugh

William Boyd by Ian Carr

CONTENTS

Acknowledgements 9

One	Introduction. William Boyd, Pathologist and Weaver of Words	11
Two	A Portsoy Boyhood	13
Three	Student in Auld Reekie	27
Four	The English Midlands: a Start in Pathology	52
Five	Ypres — The Nightingale and the Guns	64
Six	Prairie Professor	72
Seven	Halfway	95
Eight	Papers, Books and Words	115
Nine	The Zenith and the Shadow	131
Ten	Evening Comes	153

Notes 175
Appendix 1 Curriculum Vitae — William Boyd 1885-1979 179
Appendix 2 The Golden Chain: The Revisions of Boyd's Books 181
Appendix 3 Bibliography 183
Index 189

*In fond memory of my father,
C.R. Carr,
who also walked by the Menin Gate*

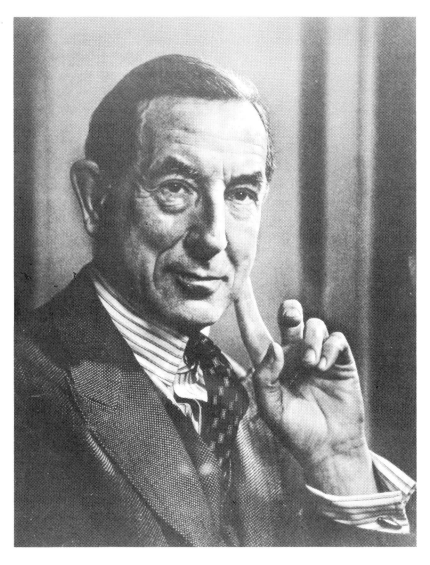

William Boyd, the mature professor. (Copyright, by permission of Karsh of Ottawa)

Acknowledgements

I thank many of Boyd's former pupils, friends and colleagues for their memories; the librarians and archivists of the Universities of Edinburgh, Manitoba, Toronto and British Columbia, of the Toronto Academy of Medicine, of the Royal College of Surgeons, Edinburgh and of Portsoy, Scotland.

In particular, I am grateful to Cleone Stoloff for Boyd's personal correspondence, photograph album, and Commonplace Book, and her recollections; to Dr. Fleming McConnell and Mr. Ian Boyd for family recollections and pictures; to Dr. E.J. Bowmer for letters between Boyd and Dr. F.W. Wiglesworth. These materials will be added to the extensive collection of his original handwritten manuscripts, and other memorabilia, to be deposited in the Fisher Library of the University of Toronto as the "William Boyd Papers" or will be displayed in the University of Manitoba Medical Library. To Dr. John Barrie who entertained me for hours with his memories; to Dr. Jan Hoogstraaten who generously gave me unpublished material on the history of pathology in the University of Manitoba, partly derived from archival material now lost; to Dr. David Hardwick of the University of British Columbia and Dr. Malcolm Silver of the University of Toronto for their help. Drs. Robert Beamish, Drummond Bowden, James Henderson and Keith Sandiford, and Mrs. Marie Crookston and Katharine Weiss generously spent time on criticism of the text. I owe an especial debt to Professor Audrey Kerr, University of Manitoba Medical Library.

—— Chapter 1 ——

Introduction — William Boyd, Pathologist and Weaver of Words

WILLIAM BOYD died in 1979, full of years and honours, the most successful pathology teacher of his time, one of the greatest medical writers and teachers of the twentieth century, a figure of distinction in Canadian medical history.

Boyd was born in Portsoy in the northeast of Scotland on 21 June 1885, and trained in medicine in Edinburgh. After graduation he worked in mental hospitals in the English Midlands and for a short time as a pathologist in Wolverhampton. He was appointed Professor of Pathology in the University of Manitoba in 1915 but spent a brief eventful spell in the front line in Flanders as a medical officer before taking up his appointment in Winnipeg. In twenty-two years in Winnipeg he attained a major international reputation as a writer of texts on pathology, the scientific basis of the understanding of disease. He became Professor and Head of Pathology in the University of Toronto in 1937. After retiring from Toronto in 1951 he spent three years as the first Professor of Pathology in the new medical school of the University of British Columbia. His textbooks, noted for their readability, brought him fame and financial profit. He was renowned for his skill as a speaker and teacher, but if his tongue was silver his pen was golden. He died on March 10, 1979. (Please see Appendix 1)

He left behind him monuments more enduring than bronze — books which ran into many editions. They influenced innumerable medical students and made him famous throughout the medical world. His neat, confident figure and Scottish accent were well known in the smaller world of pathologists. He was talking, always talking, often emphasizing a point with a twitch of an eyebrow, often a cigarette in hand. He would have wished to be remembered as he was in his prime, photographed by Karsh.

People record their lives in what they leave behind — memories, friends, pupils, buildings, books, children. Part of Boyd's life is easy to find in his writings and, where possible, I have used his own words. The rest has been pieced together from his friends' recollections, and by visiting the places where he grew up, was educated and worked. Often I have been tempted to write more discursively about the background, because Boyd lived in interesting times and places. The constraints of the publishers have kept me in the narrow way and the references to sources relatively brief.

I met and heard him speak only once, when he was an old man, frail, yet with residual sparkle. As his biographer, I have been entranced walking in his footsteps, reading his letters, talking to his friends, listening to those who did not like him and watching a videotape of the man in old age. My enquiries started without the bias of a pupil. I did not read his books until recently, but chose to write about him because he spent his most productive days in the medical school in which I work. I felt a kinship with this Scotsman who spent two decades on the Canadian prairie yet still dreamt of the hills. It is a rare privilege to speak with a ghost, and see a little into another soul.

Chapter 2

A Portsoy Boyhood

THE PLACE where one spends one's first few years leaves an indelible stamp. Boyd was born in 1885 in Portsoy on the Moray coast of Scotland into the Free Kirk manse, the last of six children, of whom one had died young. The certificate reads, "Born 1885 June Twenty-first 7h30m a.m. Free Church Manse, Portsoy of Dugald Cameron Boyd Free Church Clergyman and Eliza Marion Boyd M.S. Butcher Date and place of marriage 1867 May 8th Mahableshwar-Bombay." His advent so late in a marriage might have been a little unpremeditated, but that was not unusual then. His father, Dugald Cameron Boyd, was born in Glasgow in 1832 and studied for the ministry at the University of St. Andrews and at New College, Edinburgh. He entered the ministry shortly after the Disruption of the Free Church from the established Presbyterian Church of Scotland, an event that aroused passions to a height today reserved only for pop singers or hockey stars. He chose the Free Church, "the wee kirk, the free kirk, the kirk wi'oot the steeple", as opposed to "the auld kirk, the cauld kirk, the kirk wi'oot the people". The choice bespoke his enthusiastic evangelical outlook.

After ordination he was called to minister to the English-speaking congregation in Madras. The family tale is that Dugald Boyd, a well-set, handsome young man, had fallen in love with the daughter of a promi-

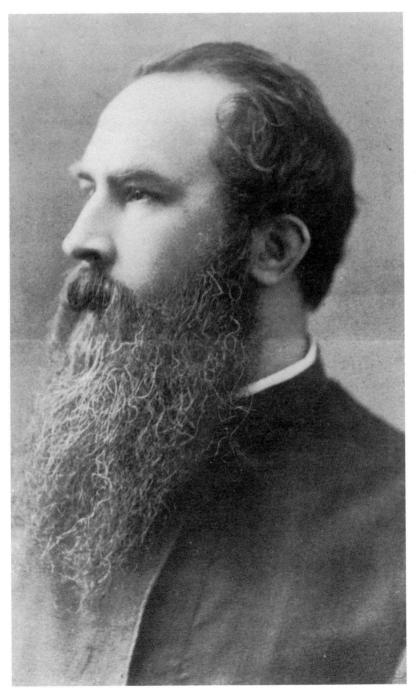
Dugald Boyd in 1867

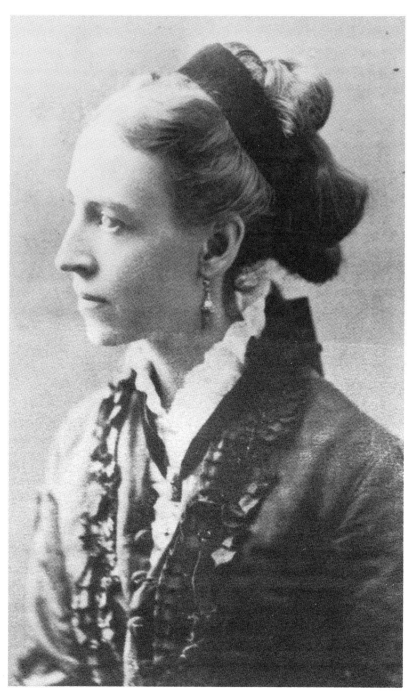

Elizabeth Boyd in 1867

nent British Liberal politician. She reciprocated the feeling passionately, but her parents were not enthusiastic, and arranged that the holy young swain be sent to a distant part of the Empire. Soon after he arrived in India a dreamily beautiful young woman, Eliza Marion Butcher, daughter of a well-off military man, walked into his church. Shortly afterwards, in 1867, they were married. He resigned in 1877 and returned to settle in Portsoy in 1879, staying there until 1895, when he became Secretary of the Anglo-Indian Evangelical Society. He died of tuberculosis in 1898.

Portsoy

Much of the Portsoy that Dugald Boyd knew is still there. Caravans (camper-trailers), street lights, and council houses do not obscure the core of grey stone and narrow, winding streets. The cottages of the fishermen, the fisher-row, lie beside the harbour well protected by strong stone piers.

A village with a considerable history, in 1550 Portsoy was created a Burgh of Barony by Mary of Guise, Regent for Mary Queen of Scots; this gave an already established fishing and trading community an enhanced standing. In 1881 the population was about 2000. A small boy would have seen a harbour full of fishing boats, some picturesque Zulu open yawls which had filled Scottish harbours in the 1870s, some herring drifters and a few of the early steam trawlers. The fishing generated work on shore: coopering, salting, kippering and packing. It was seasonal because the boats and the fishwives followed the herring shoals all the way round the Scottish coast, from Banff to Kinlochbervie to Campbeltown and further south. Fishwives with their creels, commonplace on the streets, took day-return tickets on the train to sell their wares up-country.

As well as sea fishing, there was salmon stake-net fishing. The economy until 1750 had been mediaeval, but by 1810 enclosure was complete; the linen industry had been prosperous in the previous century and meanwhile other industries had developed in the village. In 1890 a young lad would have seen a foundry which made capstans, a shipyard which built small fishing boats, a rope walk, a mill powered by the mill-dam on Loch Soy, a bone meal plant, a distillery and a quarry. There were several banks and insurance agencies, the usual butcher's, baker's and grocer's shops, and, important in a candle-lit world, a tallow chandlery.

The streets were narrow, part cobbled, elsewhere rutted and muddy.

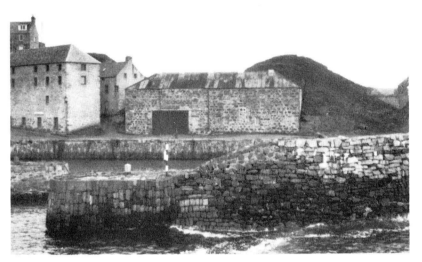

Portsoy Harbour in 1988 (Author's photograph)

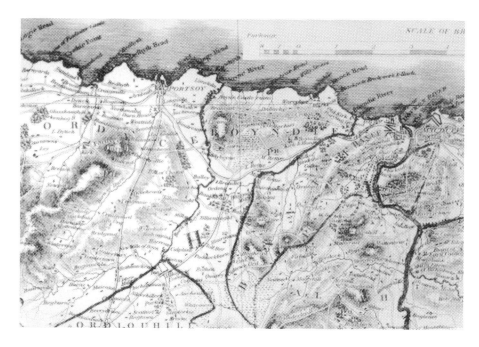

A map of Portsoy and the surrounding areas of Banffshire, as it was in 1800

On his way as he went to school, young William Boyd would walk beside fishwives with their creels, pass lines of pack-horses or carts headed to and from the harbour, and schoolchildren, barefoot in the summer. "Foggie Loan Johnnie" the packman went on his way to the farm towns. The market was held weekly, and there the gypsies could be seen offering to tinker pots. The language of the streets was the rich Buchan dialect, the language of Charles Murray and the bothy* balladeers — far from standard English. "Man, Dod, dae ye min' fan we coupit yer faither's cairt intae the Herbour on Hogmanay nicht?" (Do you remember when we pushed your father's cart into the Harbour on New Year's Eve?) In an educated household the young grew up bilingual.

The railway took a while to reach Portsoy. The Banff, Portsoy and Strathisla Railway, started in 1859, had amalgamated into the Great North of Scotland Railway in 1867, but the loop was completed only in 1886; the line reached Portsoy Harbour slightly later. From about 1870 the turnpike roads had been good in the North; Royal Mail coaches ran from Portsoy to Aberdeen and Inverness.

Kirks and Pubs
A son of the manse would have gone to kirk twice on the Sabbath. As he walked up the steps into the kirk, he would have seen the parade of the "unco guid", men in top hats and frock coats, women in lace-trimmed tippets and ostrich-feathered bonnets. There was a kirk for most tastes: the Church of Scotland and the Free Church of Scotland, built at the Disruption in 1843 and rebuilt with a steeple in 1869. This was where Dugald Boyd ministered from 1879 to 1895; it is now the Church of Scotland, "The West Kirk". The Free Presbyterian Church, the Episcopal Church and the Roman Catholic Church completed the roster. The Free Church, more than the others, was the Church of the predestined elect: Calvinistic, strict and teetotal.

There were sixteen pubs — the Star, the Thistle, the Ship, and so on; the sight of a drunk man in the streets was no rarer than in similar fishing villages in the 1940s. The pubs were usually full, but drunkenness was intermittently mitigated by concentrated doses of divine mercy in the form of evangelical revivals. A revival was usual after a disaster, as when the ship "Annie" collided and sank on 20 January 1887; eight

---

*bothy — a humble room or cottage where unmarried farm labourers are housed.

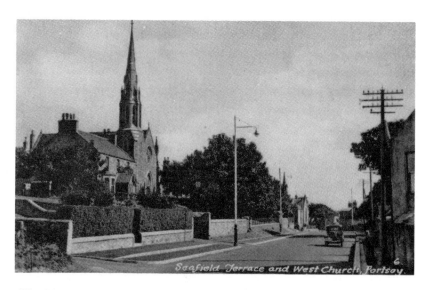

The West Kirk, Portsoy, as seen in a postcard illustration, taken in the 1930s

local men died leaving four widows and twenty orphans. In a society devoid of systematic social security, "cold as charity" was a merited simile. After the great gale of 1893, religious revival swept the fishing villages: "Tibby, your Johnny was saved in Portsoy last night." went the word. During such revivals, divine mercy must have been sloshing around the corridors of a Free Kirk manse. The young Boyd must have been marinated in the nurture and admonition of the Lord. The public morality was that of John Calvin. Stools of repentance had last been heard of in the parish in 1624, and acts against witches in 1670. However, they were still folk memories.

Death Walked Openly
Health was that of a third world community; water went short in the summer, sanitation was largely dry, and the night soil wagons went their rounds. There was no control of bovine tuberculosis. Scarlet fever, diphtheria, typhoid and, less often, typhus and smallpox were epidemic. In the 1880s, anaesthesia was only a little over thirty years old and older folk could remember the horrors of pre-anaesthetic surgery. The germ theory of disease was new, and antiseptic surgery, introduced in 1867, was not accepted by all surgeons. Poverty, poor housing, malnutrition and death in childbirth were common. In Portsoy the Campbell Hospital was opened in 1904 to cope with epidemic disease. Death walked more openly in those days, and the fear of death and of the Lord were indeed regarded as the beginning of wisdom.

Most people could read, even if they read only the local newspaper, the "Tammy", and knew of happenings in the wider world. Folk from the district, poor and rich, went off to serve and die in, or return rich from the farthest corners of Victoria's Empire. Gladstone fought Disraeli at the hustings and intelligent discussions of Gladstone's Midlothian campaign appeared in local newspapers. It is fair to assume that opinion on Disraeli in the local pubs was as corrosive as that on Thatcher, his Conservative successor, a century later.

The time and place conditioned young William Boyd. It was not a bad place to be a wee boy. Education in the area was of a relatively high standard for the time because of significant bequests which augmented teachers' salaries in the area.

We know little detail of Boyd's childhood and can only surmise what life was like in the manse. Perhaps the best place to recapture the flavour

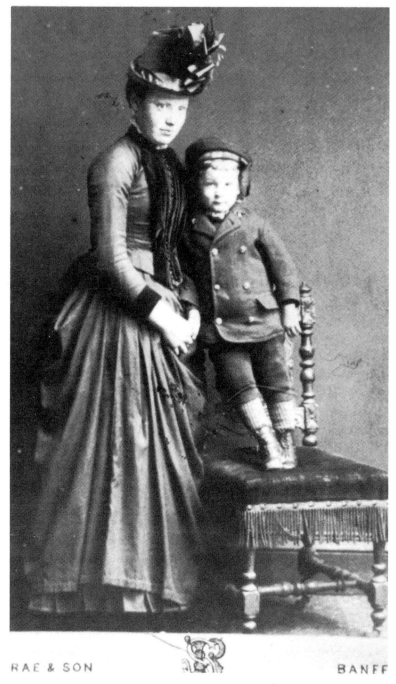
William Boyd and his mother

of a boyhood in a Free Kirk manse of the period is in Alistair Phillips' *My Uncle George*, set in Fearn in Ross-shire a little further up the Scottish coast. Bread was home baked in a coal-fired oven and milk straight from the cow was unpasteurized. Fish, usually herring, was prominent in the diet. Breakfast consisted of salted but unsweetened porridge. Religion was ever present — a firm if not stern religion in which right was right and punishment certain. Minor corporal punishment was accepted in rearing children. A spanking — a skelpit leathering — quickly solved many problems.

Free education was universal in Scotland at this time, but many, particularly rural children, left school at twelve years of age. The stratification of social classes was less than in England. The choice of primary school in Portsoy was limited to a dame school, run by gentlewomen for a modest fee, and the local primary school. There is no information as to young William's initial schooling.

We have pictures of the boy himself with his mother, who was well educated and highly literate and had a great influence on him, encouraging particularly his love of literature. We see him, the youngest, the "shakings of the poke", in the midst of his family. The bearded patriarch was old to have a son Will's age; his siblings ten years or more older were often more like uncles and an aunt. They scattered like thistledown round the world, but later he was to have good contacts with them. Herbert (1868-1936) practised law in Wetaskiwin, Alberta. Hugh (1869-1895) died young. Arnold (1870-1958) became a minister, for a long time in Naranderra, New South Wales. Guy (1872-1930) farmed in Thetford, Ontario. Winifred (1875-1952), of whom he was very fond, became a school teacher in the north of England, but had recurrent major psychiatric illness.

We know even less about Boyd's life from about 1894, when the family left Portsoy for Glasgow. His father suffered from pulmonary tuberculosis from which he died in 1898. Between 1895 and 1898 William attended Glasgow Academy, then as now an excellent school for the upper class. The Boyds lived first at 11 Albion Street and then (1896-8) at 3 Queen Margaret Crescent, a prosperous middle-class area. Presumably his mother's family helped defray expenses.

We have a record that thereafter he attended Trent Academy in Derbyshire, but there is no detail, except that he kept to the end of his days the leather-bound prize books he won there. He was probably sent to boarding school, a niece speculates, to avoid being brought up entirely by women. The end result was a young man, if not of the upper crust, at least above the middle.

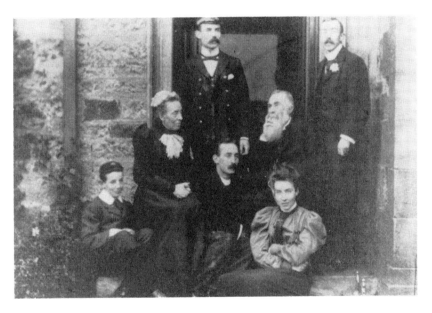

The Boyd family in the 1890s; William seated at the left

Family Register.

Dugald Cameron Boyd and Eliza Marian Butcher were married at Mahableshwur, Bombay Presidency, 8th. May 1867 —

Herbert Cameron, their first-born child, was born in Bombay ——— 2d. June 1868.

Hugh Arthur, their second child, was born in Bombay - 27th. Nov. 1869. Died in Cuttack, Orissa - 11th April 1895.

Arnold, their third child, was born in Bombay — 17th. Sept. 1870. Died in Leven, Fifeshire, 14th March 1958

Guy Westwood, their fourth child, was born in Bombay. 19. Aug/72. Died in Strathroy, Ont. 22 Aug. 1932

Winifred, their fifth child, was born in Bombay, 3d. April 1875. Died in Edinburgh. Feb 5. 1952

William, their sixth child, was born in Portsoy - 21st. June 1885. Died in Toronto, 10 March, 1979.

Dugald Cameron Boyd died at Dalry, Ayrshire. 3rd December, 1898.

Eliza Marian Boyd died at N. Shields. 31 Dec. 191

Boyd family register, in the front of the family Bible

Chapter 3
A Student in Auld Reekie

WE MEET Boyd, aged 18, as a medical student in Edinburgh in 1903. His university record shows that he had attained in October 1902 higher mathematics, lower Latin, English and French, and was exempted from examination in physics in 1903. His school background was adequate, but not distinguished. He went to university in a society which had just been shaken by the South African War. In the background during his student and early graduate days were the political rivalries, the diplomatic incidents and the arms race that led to World War I. In 1903 there was little awareness that the days of the Long Peace were numbered.

Edinburgh was indeed Auld Reekie, a smoky place through whose "wynds and vennels" whistled at once the caller breezes of the North Sea, and the residual winds of a senescent but not yet moribund Calvinism. The winds must have blown hard for the son of a Free Church manse, because the Disruption was still within the memory of older people. The grey Edinburgh tenements do not encourage frivolous thought. The influence of the church was strong and many Scottish children went through a conflict which almost might be termed religious melancholia, before the age of ten. Some carried their guilt and fears into adult life.

On a Sunday morning people of all ages streamed to church in twos and threes, in family squadrons, or in crocodile formation, feet clacking

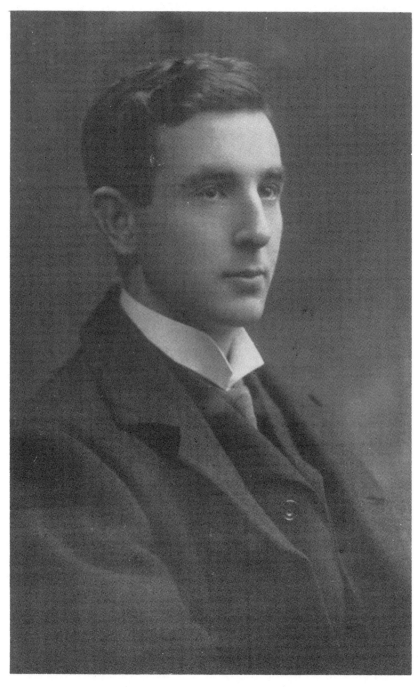

William Boyd in his Edinburgh days

on the cobbles. Women still wore long dresses and usually wore their hair coiled, wound into a teapot handle and secured on the crown of the head. On the sabbath there was little wheeled traffic other than an occasional horse cab or doctor's brougham.

A popular preacher had the attraction that is now found in a film star, and was a wonderful influence in the church. The great word in the church was "mission" — whether abroad or at home. Some medical students were heavily involved in home missions and visited sad invalid children, stricken by tuberculosis, paralysis or feeble-mindedness.

University and Medical School
The University was and always had been closely bound to the City Corporation, which had considerable powers of patronage. The medical school dominated the University, especially since Sir William Turner, the former Professor of Anatomy, had succeeded a long line of divines and philosophers as Principal. Crum Brown, Professor of Chemistry, an ancient alchemist in skull-cap and long gown, was a polymath of a kind now unknown; he had been a candidate also for professorships in Greek and mathematics. From 1903 to 1906 Boyd sat under Daniel John Cunningham, Professor of Anatomy and author of a major text and a dissecting manual. The study of gross anatomy still dominated medical education. Although body-snatchers, the "sack 'em up" men, were gone, not a few medical students would obtain skulls as did one of Boyd's contemporaries, Isabel Hutton, from a country graveyard. Physiology was taught by Edward Schafer, a leader in the field. Boyd did well, obtaining medals in practical anatomy and physiology. Pathology was taught by W.S. Greenfield, whose neuropathology text later became famous. Greenfield did not impress the young Boyd nor for that matter did Boyd make an impression as a student of pathology. Attendance at autopsies for six months was mandatory.

We have a very good idea just what Boyd studied in pathology from the meticulously kept notebook of his classmate, Alexander Gibson, which is in the Medical Library in Winnipeg. There was much morbid anatomy and bacteriology, but as yet little immunology; viruses had been described but were still unimportant in the curriculum. The evangelical hand was felt in strange places; the Professor of Pathology (Greenfield) led teams of students on evangelical missions to save souls in such pagan places as darkest Glasgow.

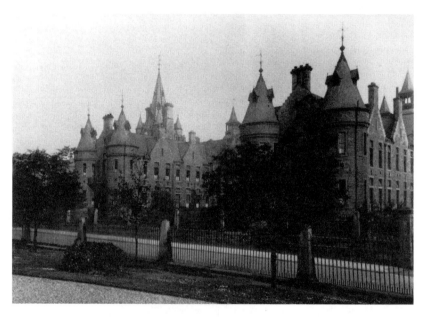

Royal Infirmary, Edinburgh, in the early 1900s (Courtesy of Edinburgh University Library)

The medical course lasted for five years — 100 lectures each in anatomy and in chemistry and 50 each in physics, zoology and botany. It was the day of the lecture; medical students had need of long ears, ready pens and broad rumps. The defect in the Edinburgh undergraduate training of the day was, perhaps, lack of clinical material. Unkind graduates of other schools said that their Edinburgh counterparts knew everything but could do nothing.

Boyd had two classmates who were later to be important in his life — Alexander Gibson and J.C.B. Grant. Gibson had been an extraordinarily bright student in the Faculty of Arts, and in Medicine had repeated the performance. He graduated first in the year, with 1st Class Honours and the Eccles Scholarship, the coveted award given to the top-ranking student in the year. Grant graduated with 2nd Class Honours. Boyd, though a successful student who never failed an examination, gained an ordinary degree. Gibson became Professor of Anatomy in the Manitoba Medical School and was later to bring Boyd and Grant to Winnipeg.

Edinburgh was steeped in Listerian tradition. Joseph Lister had proved the value of antiseptic surgery in Glasgow in 1867 through the use of the carbolic spray, but he moved to Edinburgh not long after, where he changed the surgical world from his Edinburgh Chair. The memory of James Young Simpson, the great anaesthetist was still fresh. People could remember when surgery had meant agony; women in particular equated childbirth with prolonged, unrelieved pain. Simpson's funeral procession through the streets of Edinburgh in 1870 resembled the obsequies of a monarch rather than the interment of a physician. It is difficult for us to realize what it was like to have walked so closely behind such immortals.

Clinical teaching was in the hands of the honorary staff*; the student chose which "chief" to work under. Antiseptic surgery was in full swing, but of course there were neither sulphonamides nor systemic antibiotics. Each student was assigned three cases in the winter, and two in the summer, and wrote up a complete record of history and clinical findings. The student did the elementary laboratory tests in the "side

---

*When Boyd was a medical student, no patient in a teaching hospital received a bill from a physician; the physician's reward for teaching and looking after patients for nothing was his enhanced reputation in the eyes of the community on which he depended for his professional income.

room" and later, in the evening between seven and eight-thirty, dressed the surgical wounds. Tuberculous glands in the neck were common; it required considerable surgical finesse to dissect them off the carotid arteries. Thomas Annandale, Professor of Clinical Surgery, did not quite believe in Listerian antisepsis. He merely washed his hands before an operation, but he could amputate a leg in two minutes. John Chiene, a faithful disciple of Lister, was Professor of Surgery. He was a godly man who used the scalpel only when he had to, and preached the virtues of total abstinence from alcohol, a controversial view in a society polarized on temperance.

The Professor of Medicine, John Wyllie, a bachelor, wore a flower in his buttonhole as he did his ward round. Sir Thomas Fraser, Professor of Materia Medica, held his clinics in a lecture theatre. He treated pneumonia with large doses of digitalis, which helped prevent any complicating heart failure but did little for the infection. The Professor of Pathology, Dr. Greenfield, had charge of wards and taught on patients by the bedside. There was separate teaching for women students.

Student Life
Boyd stayed in Lonsdale Terrace. The records of his own student days are patchy — a photographic album, a hiking diary, a few later reminiscences. The album is bound in standard green leathercloth 9.5 by 7 inches. It shows Arran, Garelochhead and Loch Long, Arrochar, Ben Nevis, Skiddaw, Derwentwater. The hiking diary, a little soft-bound book, labelled "Hiking Diary W. Boyd", was started on 2 September 1903 and records trips to Cairngorm, Snowdon, Great Gable and Goat Fell. Their climbing was the real thing, often in winter with ice axes on snow-covered summits. Other pictures show young men on a fishing boat, or picnicking with unidentified young ladies.

Alec Gibson was a frequent companion, as noted in Boyd's hiking diary:

> The one thing I taught him in our undergraduate days was rock climbing, and on Saturday afternoons we used to bicycle to the Salisbury Crags adjoining Arthur's Seat just outside Edinburgh, and climb those vertical cliffs with the safeguard of an alpine rope. Our greatest thrill was when we managed to do the climb called

Extract from Boyd's climbing diary; HCB is Hector Cameron Boyd, his eldest brother, and AG is Alexander Gibson.

> 29. <u>Sgur Banachdich & Loch Coruisk.</u>
> 3rd July. 1908.
> F.G., C.M., A.G., & W.B.
>
> | | |
> |---|---|
> | Glen Brittle | 11.30.p.m. |
> | Top of Banachdich | 3.0 – 4.20. |
> | Bathe in Coruisk & Breakfast | 7.45 – 8.30. |
> | Sleep by Coruisk | 9.15 – 10.45 |
> | Bathe in Scavaig | 11.15 |
> | Left Coruisk | 1.0 |
> | Lunch | 1.30 – 2.0. |
> | Top of Druim Hain, watching the Coolin | 2.50 – 3.30 |
> | Sligachan | 5.45 |
> | Portree | 10.30 |

Extract from Boyd's climbing diary

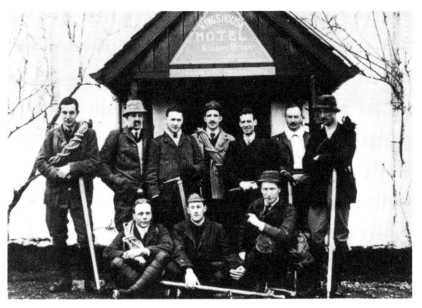

A climbing party (Boyd, back row left) at the Kingshouse Hotel, about 1908

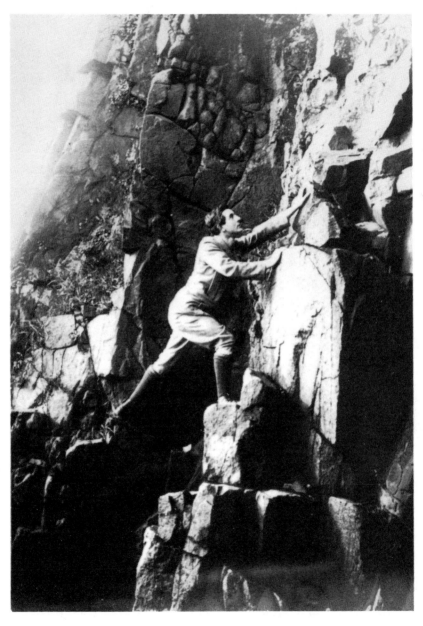

William Boyd climbing, as a student, probably on the Salisbury Crags, Edinburgh

the Cracked Slabs. When we struggled to the top, Alec stood on his head in triumph.

When the result of the second-year examination came out (Alec with first-class honours, I with none), we started out to bicycle south to the English Lake District, where we spent a heavenly two weeks, walking and climbing.

A contemporary, John Lechler, who came up to Edinburgh University to study medicine in 1902, and who lived to a similarly ripe age, has left a vivid picture of life as a medical student in the Edinburgh of that day. On his first day as a student he went to the YMCA, which served among other things as a student lodgings office, and was given an address in Cumberland Street. He shared lodgings with three others and paid less than fifteen shillings a week for a room and three meals a day. Breakfast was a large plate of porridge and a halfpenny "bap" (bread roll). They walked to and from Teviot Place, the medical school, coming home for lunch.

It is always difficult to assess the cost of living in another time. The middle class were comfortably off but the poor were really poor, poorer than the poorest in Scotland today. A made-to-measure suit cost three guineas. A pair of shoes ten shillings. Milk was a penny a pint, and bread twopence for a large loaf. Whisky was half-a-crown a bottle and tobacco twopence an ounce. Woodbine cigarettes were five a penny and postage a penny. Most students were quite poor. "Meal Monday" came in the middle of the term when traditionally the student would go home and replenish his "kist"* of meal. Supper at the Union (the students' club) might be "cockie-leekie and fine minced collops"**. Most students stayed in lodgings or "digs" whose owners, maiden ladies or widows, eked out a living by taking one or two lodgers. There were a few "chronics" who failed examinations regularly and remained students for many years. Relaxation was obtained by playing rugby at Craiglockhart or rowing on the river.

The Union held regular debates at which Boyd learned to speak in public. He admitted later that he was so shy at first that he went to several debates intending to speak but was too tongue-tied to open his mouth.

---

* Storage box, usually of wood
**Soup made of a cock and leek; collops are ground meat

There were five o'clock concerts given by the students — here, too, he must have learned to shed some inhibitions because as an older student he was often on his feet to lead a chorus at a dinner or a party. On a Saturday night the students would dance on the newly sprung floor to the strains of "The Blue Danube" and "The Merry Widow". Perhaps it was here that Boyd learned to dance; he enjoyed dancing till late in life. There were London plays at the Lyceum Theatre (cheap seats sixpence) and there were musical comedies and grand operas.

The Home Mission in the Cowgate established by the Edinburgh Medical Missionary Society was set up in an old whisky shop. The poor were seen free of charge; there was one resident doctor; and twelve students who did home visits. The mission, opened by David Livingstone, provided food tickets and lodgings for the poor. There was no form of health insurance and the honorary physician (the physician was almost always male) looked after the poor for nothing while he made a living from the ills of the rich. The many Edinburgh poor sought help in the Cowgate where the students' medical experience ranged from domiciliary midwifery to attending the victims of attempted murder or the aftermath of murder itself.

Examinations ruled a student's life. Chemistry and physics, botany and zoology in the first year. Anatomy, physiology and materia medica at the end of third year; pathology at the end of fourth year. The Great Hall of the old Adam building with its huge dome was used for professional examinations. Male medical students were taught in the late-Victorian medical school building next to the Royal Infirmary.

Clinical Teaching
Isabel Hutton, another contemporary, remembered her student days vividly fifty years later. Women students went to the Medical School only for examinations but were taught in the Surgeons' Hall in Nicholson Street. Students spent two years as surgical dressers in the Royal Infirmary. Classes were held in the large lecture theatre where there were "great semicircles of shabby brown wooden seats rising steeply upwards towards the roof and a small semi-circle of plain deal floor". Surgical clinics were held twice weekly and, despite Lister, asepsis was not yet absolute. In some theatres, practice was still antiseptic rather than aseptic; instruments were boiled and then placed in one-in-twenty carbolic and handed to the surgeon by well-scrubbed but ungloved hands.

Students learned to bandage, to put on plaster casts and jackets, and to prepare splints for operations and emergencies.

Unsupervised students gave chloroform from a round, dark blue, twelve-ounce bottle, the stab end of a large safety pin being thrust into its neck, thus propping up the stopper and allowing the fluid to escape in a liberal stream onto a folded face towel. It was not unknown for the surgeon to hear the words, "The patient's stopped breathing, Sir." The new gauze-covered metal masks with a small chloroform-dropper bottle came in later. Students on casualty duty saw life in the raw particularly on Saturday nights.

As Seniors in the fourth and fifth year they attended the medical wards to learn the details of medical and neurological examination. The medical wards by comparison with the surgical were tranquil places where the pace was often set by the elderly nursing sister. Two elegant and learned physicians would walk into their ward at precisely the same hour in the morning to visit their patients and to teach the assembled students. Each wore a top hat, frock coat, sponge-bag trousers and black kid gloves, having come on foot from their consulting rooms in the West End of Edinburgh. Their monaural stethoscopes would often be carried inside their top hats. They departed at one o'clock having timed their entrance and exit to avoid interrupting the ward routine.

The students studied pathology in the fourth year and learned to cut and stain microscope sections to satisfy Professor Greenfield, a severe examiner who had the reputation of failing candidates many times over. In materia medica they learned to make pills, fold powders, make up mixtures and write prescriptions in Latin.

Boyd wrote much later: "One spring day in Edinburgh, the Third Professional Examinations came to an end. For months I had not opened what you might call a decent book. The last quiz was held that morning. After lunch I drew my chair to an open window, lit a pipe, and began to read of d'Artagnan, riding on that sorry nag of his up the streets of Meung — my first introduction to the Musketeers."

A Coo and a Coontess
The Professor of Midwifery, Halliday Croom, was a tall, spare, grand seigneur in morning dress with pince-nez spectacles protected from crashing on the floor by a black ribbon attached at the other end to his lapel. Spicing his lectures with Rabelaisian anecdotes, he related in broad Scots:

"D'ye ken that the only difference between a coo and a coontess is the curve of Carus [the pelvic curve]?" Scots physicians still spoke the vernacular because that was all many of their patients understood.

Life was especially hard for women, bearing their children with great fortitude, in or out of wedlock, in miserable hovels. Family planning was unheard of. Congenital syphilis was common. Silver nitrate was instilled into a newborn's eyes to prevent gonococcal ophthalmia.

Students attended one of the several dispensaries for the treatment of the poor — Cowgate Medical Mission or St. John's Dispensary. Edinburgh was a city where drunkenness was rife; after late-night bacchanalia which resulted in minor casualties, the vanquished would be led up the Royal Mile towards Casualty between two great Highland bobbies. The streets were old with memories, going as far back as Mary Queen of Scots.

The poor lived in very congested circumstances and many women were frightened about incest, yet medical students received no instruction on how to deal with sexual or marital problems. The nearest they came to receiving advice on counselling was to attend a course of lectures on venereal disease in the Lock Wards high up in the attics of the Royal Infirmary.

Patients with venereal diseases were treated punitively, without sympathy or understanding, as befitted "sinners". Those who could pay, discreetly consulted a specialist in sexually transmitted disease who linked his special skill to dermatology — a blessed protection against discovery for wealthy sinners. All public venereal disease clinics were held in a bare brown room with a rough wooden floor, and patients were examined on deal trestle tables. Urethral infusions of silver nitrate were used in the treatment of gonorrhoea in men, and syphilis was treated with large quantities of mercury and bismuth. Urethral strictures were dilated by the passage of bougies. This procedure was painful, particularly in the hands of inexperienced students. The end result was frequently serious trauma to the urethra. The whole procedure might have been devised by Calvin as a prophylactic against sin. Women patients wore drab, ugly uniforms and their hair in plaits. Apart from an occasional concert by students, nothing was done to amuse or instruct the patients.

Patients with infectious disease were segregated in separate wards round which students, dressed in protective mother hubbards, used to follow the physician. In those days children were encouraged to con-

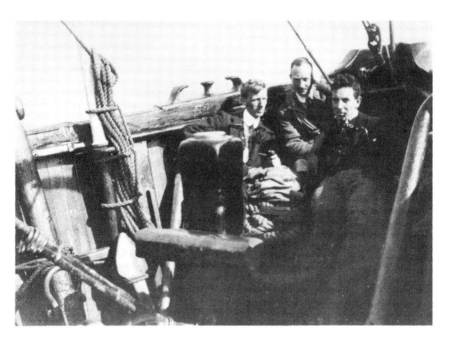

Over the sea to Skye, past the enchanted islands (Boyd with pipe)

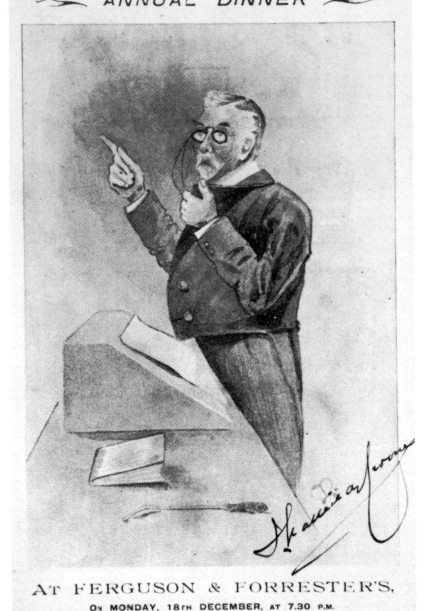

An Edinburgh University medical students' dinner menu in 1906

[Signatures]

Students' Chorus after "Alma Mater."

Gaudeamus igitur, juvenes dum sumus,
Gaudeamus igitur, juvenes dum sumus,
Post jucundam juventutem, post molestam senectutem,
Nos habebit humus, nos habebit humus.

Vivat Academia, vivant Professores,
Vivat Academia, vivant Professores,
Vivant Anni Quarti Studentes Medicinæ,
Semper sint in flore, semper sint in flore!

[Signatures]

From the same menu. Earth has indeed now received them, but once they rejoiced.

tract fevers — measles, chicken pox or mumps. It was hoped that a courageous confrontation might stay the reaper's scythe. Training in dealing with mental illness was remarkably adequate; the neurologist and the psychiatrist had not yet so completely gone their separate ways.

As a clinical student, Boyd was particularly attracted to Byron Bramwell, a master teacher, devoted to neurology and psychiatry, to whom he was to dedicate his first medical book.

Medical training ended with the dreaded "Finals". Boyd wrote much later, in 1931, "And again when the Final Examinations came to a close after six weeks of torture, four of us got on the night train from Edinburgh to Oban and sailed the whole of that perfect June day over the sea to Skye past the enchanted islands." It was an experience he remembered all his days. In 1965, in a Memorial Lecture dedicated to his friend Alec Gibson, he described how on

> the evening of the day on which the results of that purgatory of six weeks, the final examination, were published (with the same spread of honours as before), Alec and I and four non-medical friends boarded the 10 p.m. train for Oban in the Western Highlands. We had never heard of sleeping cars, so we each rented a pillow for sixpence and slept soundly till 4 a.m. when we reached Oban on the twentieth of June. At 6 a.m. we were on the steamer sailing over the sea to Skye. As we lay on the deck in the glorious sunshine all thought of those terrible weeks faded from our memory. On landing in the evening there was a mere 10-mile walk to a crofter's cottage in Glen Brittle, carrying on our backs our baggage, together with a tent for sleeping, for a two weeks' climbing holiday in the Black Coolins.
>
> Next day was the 21st of June, the longest day of the year and my own birthday, and after a swim in the sea which was only 100 yards from our tent we started on our first climb. Later in the day we stood on the summit of the Coolins and looked down:
>
> And God's own profound was above us,
> Around us the mountains, beneath us the sea.
>
> Then another swim, supper in the cottage, and dreamless sleep in our tent.

It was a good way to recover from stress.

George Buchanan's Breeches
At the end of the course those who were not weeded out by the examinations graduated in the McEwan Hall Bachelor of Medicine and Chirurgery garbed in fur-edged magenta hoods and mortar boards.

> How proud my mien when I heard the Dean
> Proclaim my name and station.
> How swells my heart as I play my part
> In this great graduation.
> How pleasant the tap of the velvet cap
> Which old tradition teaches
> Was made from the rear of a half-used pair
> Of George Buchanan's breeches.

The verses, by Douglas Maclagan, are quoted from Isabel Hutton's autobiography. Buchanan was a sixteenth-century philosopher, scholar and co-founder of the University of Edinburgh.

The pattern is recognizable to the Scottish medical graduate of today, and not strange to anyone who has trained in medicine. The medicine Boyd learned had advanced considerably in theory in fifty years. Bacteriology was an established science and the cause of many bacterial diseases known, but there were still few curative drugs. People died of pneumonia, diabetes, pernicious anaemia and tuberculosis as they always had. Syphilis was a major cause of cardiovascular disease and kept the mental hospitals full. The Wassermann reaction to detect it was new, and Salvarsan to treat it came only in 1910.

Boyd graduated on the 24th July 1908, without ever having failed an examination, but without particular distinction either.

After graduation the clever and the fortunate became house physicians and surgeons, unpaid but with free board, lodging and laundry. Others went straight into general practice and a rather better living, but a hospital appointment was essential if advancement in the profession was a young man's goal. In the hierarchical world of a Scottish medical school the doors of preferment may have been closed a little more tightly to one who had not been house physician to "the Professor". But Boyd had the advantage of working first at Edinburgh Royal Infirmary under

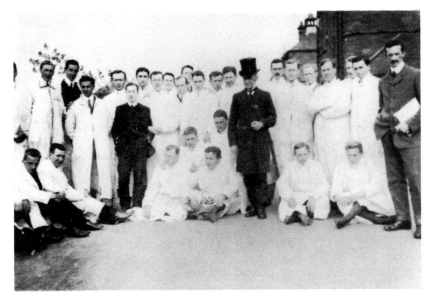

Royal Infirmary, Edinburgh — house medical staff 1909

Byron Bramwell as clinical assistant from 1 October 1908 to 31 March 1909, and then to 30 September 1909 as his resident physician. Bramwell, later knighted, was a commanding figure as a clinical teacher and the author of a voluminious text on neurology.

Boyd's minister asked one Sunday evening if he would apply for a job in Derby Borough Asylum. Perhaps because of his sister's history of mental illness, Boyd, already interested in mental disease, said yes.

As the slender, good-looking young man, five foot nine or so, climbed on the train for Derby, he had an adequate but not outstanding record behind him. He had lost much of his shyness, he talked well and mixed well socially. Leaving his own medical school so early almost certainly barred him from an academic career within it. His steps may already have been pointed far west. By chance he had made in Alexander Gibson the right friend to help him in that direction, and to eminence.

The Commonplace Book

Boyd kept a Commonplace Book, an unusual form of self-education. This was the earliest hint that he would produce something uncommon, and it indicated a literary drive that was to turn a pathologist into a writer. The first entry was in September 1902 and the last on 27 March 1950, but more than half of the main section was entered during his Edinburgh days.

Commonplace books are relics of an older day when time was more relaxed. Entertainment was made rather than consumed. People kept diaries in which they recorded the filling and the passing of their days. In commonplace books they recorded what they read. We are known by what we read as well as by the company we keep.

Boyd's Commonplace Book was kept during the years when the world wobbled. The Long Peace ended and the crystal of the old order was shattered. A generation died and nothing has been the same since. The Great War was followed by the Depression and Dust-Bowl days. Then the drums beat again, and soon distant feet marched into the Rhineland and then invaded Austria, Czechoslovakia and finally Poland; and the Second World War had begun.

The tradition of the Commonplace book is found in the late fifteenth and sixteenth centuries. The books were used at the time of the Renaissance as references to which one might resort during argument. The keeping of a commonplace book gradually became the hallmark of a writer

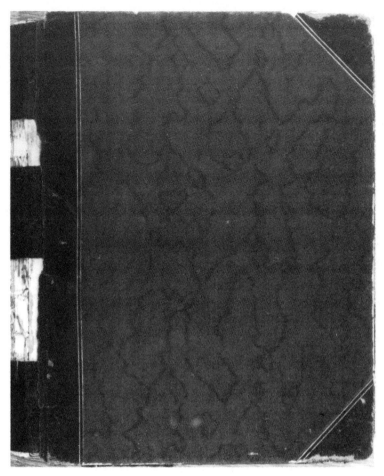

Boyd's Commonplace Book

Commonplace words

or literary man. It was, before the xerox or card index, an artificial memory. Francis Bacon advocated its use. Robert Burns, Thomas Hardy, Austin Dobson and W.H. Auden have left interesting commonplace books. Boyd was in good company.

Boyd's Commonplace Book is bound in cloth, with a leather back, now torn off, and leather corners. The inner-front flyleaf is inscribed "William Boyd" in pen and dated below 27.12.14 in pencil. The main part of the book consists of quotations in Boyd's handwriting. These are identified by author, and sometimes by book title. The first quotation, Browning's "Heroes", is dated September 1902. The main set of quotations ends on page 238, and the rest of the book, forty-five pages, is filled with further quotations. The first of these was entered in December 1906; all but two are in Boyd's handwriting. The subsidiary set is less striking than the main set, and sometimes frivolous.

The quotations deserve analysis because of what they tell about the man. One does not write out by hand a page of prose or verse unless it is agreeable or interesting to oneself. They picture the inside of the man's mind. The sources vary widely. Poetry predominates at the beginning — Robert Louis Stevenson most of all (twenty-one quotations) followed by Robert Browning (eight), Kingsley and Kipling (five each). At the end of the book there is more prose, notably quotations from John Morley and William Osler. It is a varied collection from Adam Lindsay Gordon and Euripides (in translation) to the Bible, but little Shakespeare, Milton or Wordsworth; no Keats, no Shelley; and only one quotation from Burns. There is little of what was then modern poetry, but there is prose and verse in praise of mountains, including the song of the Scottish Mountaineering Club.

The Scottish puritan tradition imbues the collection with quotations in praise of work and of what was then called purity but which might now be called repression. "Dearly beloved, I beseech you as strangers and pilgrims, abstain from fleshly lusts which war against the soul." (Jude 23). Much devotional material and prayer appear in the earlier part of the book, but not in the later. It is the collection of a widely but patchily read man, at first deeply religious, later deeply serious. "Whatsoever a man soweth, that also shall he reap." "I do not believe at all in good luck, and the man who is content to wait for a stroke of good fortune will probably wait till he has a stroke of paralysis (Treves)."

There is a devotion to work. "Work is worship" and "Do the duty which lies nearest thee which thou knowest to be a duty (Carlyle)." The devotion is cheerful. "Give us to go blithely on our business all this day . . . And grant us in the end the gift of sleep."

There is an insistence, similar to that of Osler, on worrying only about today,

> "Methinks it is the morrow, day by day
> And the coming thing alway
> Greater than things today or yesterday (Euripides: *Bacchae*)."

The book reveals a stoicism that must have served him well. "Men must endure their going hence even as their coming hither; ripeness is all." (Shakespeare: *Lear*, dated July 1904). Boyd himself went blind over seventy years later.

It is a book composed by a reader of books rather than of periodicals. There were only occasional quotations from periodicals such as the *Fortnightly Review* and the *Cornhill Magazine*.

There is a love of Scotland and its hills. "And though I think I would rather die elsewhere, yet in my heart of hearts I long to be buried in good Scots clods . . . there are no stars so lovely as Edinburgh street lamps (Stevenson)."

The academic calling is treated with a high seriousness. "Knowledge is not a couch for the curious spirit, nor a terrace for the wandering, nor a tower of state for the proud mind, nor a vantage ground for the haughty, nor a shop for profit and sale, but a storehouse for the glory of God and the endowment of mankind (Bacon)."

There are quotations that mirror his own current experiences. Louisa Alcott on the death of her mother, entered on 22.3.14, and Rupert Brooke's description of Lake Louise, dated 25.6.16. It is a reasonable bet that Boyd was off to the Rockies within six months of arriving on the prairie.

Some quotations fit his courting days. "She had a sunny nature that sought, like a flower in a dark place for the light (anon.)." "What needest with thy tribe's black tents, / Who hast the red pavilions of my heart? ("Arab Love Song", Francis Thompson)." A little later he is attracted by the art of public speaking; the book shows an interest in eloquence with quotations from Pericles, Lincoln and Bright.

He quotes the usual recipe for good writing. "A limpid style is invariably the result of hard labour (G.M. Trevelyan)." Yet Boyd's own manuscripts show only minor alterations.

There is a gap during his war service, and after it much less poetry. After 1930, the entries thin out, and after 16.2.36 there is a long gap to the last, dated 27.3.50. He was then sixty-five years old. A long life was lived between the first and the last entries in the Commonplace Book.

—— Chapter 4 ——

The English Midlands and a Start in Pathology

THE ENGLISH Midlands to a southern poet (Belloc) were sodden and unkind. To the young Boyd it was an area already partly familiar from his attendance at Trent Academy and it was to be the place where he became a pathologist. The region was smoke polluted and industrial, but the Pennines were near, where he could lift his eyes unto the hills.

Derby was a marked change from Edinburgh and not an entirely welcome one. In 1909 it was a small city of dignified brick and stone buildings, marred by grimy slums. It had a Roman heritage but there was a stronger mediaeval flavour in the layout of its narrow streets. Prince Charlie had gone no further south during his unsuccessful foray into England in the 1745 Jacobite Rebellion. Later in the 18th Century it had social and intellectual pretensions; at the Derby Assembly no lady was allowed to dance in a long white apron, and there Erasmus Darwin had founded the Philosophical Society. It had subsequently become industrialized and much of the old city had subsequently been destroyed by the advance of industrialization. Several industries flourished — textiles, notably silk, as well as china and iron. In 1908 Rolls Royce founded a new motor car factory to turn out 200 cars a year.

Derby was not a medical teaching centre, but it had some medical traditions. The Derbyshire General Infirmary, founded in 1810, was rebuilt in 1894 as the Derbyshire Royal Infirmary. There were two mental hospitals, the Derby County Asylum with about 700 patients, and the Derby Borough Asylum, which became the Kingsway Hospital. This hospital, opened in 1894, is a dignified Victorian building accommodating about 350 patients. Boyd arrived there in 1909, on completion of his house physician post at Edinburgh Royal Infirmary. The asylum of that time was a community in which many of the staff as well as all the patients lived. Those patients who were well enough worked in the gardens or at simple manufacturing tasks. It cost a little over ten shillings a week to maintain a patient.

Asylum Physician

For two years the young Dr. Boyd worked with or (more likely in the terms of the day) for Dr. S. Rutherford Macphail, an Edinburgh graduate, who was probably an acquaintance of Byron Bramwell. The hospital report for 1911 notes that he carried out his duties well. He was responsible for the initial physical examination of patients and the supervision of their long stay in hospital. There were no psychoactive drugs and therefore there was little chance of affecting the course of mental illness.

Although the life of the asylum physician was not unpleasant, it was not easy to fill medical vacancies; then, as now, these jobs were low in the medical pecking order. Salaries were not generous; the medical superintendent at the County Asylum received £250 per annum, and the junior medical officer £90. The salaries in the Borough Asylum were probably similar. At that time an average industrial wage was £80 per year. Asylum physicians usually had either free or subsidized accommodation and often free food, so that the position was not unattractive. The junior physician was expected to be available to participate in the daily activities of the hospital — the visitation by the Commissioners of Lunacy, who were responsible for maintaining standards, the visits by representatives of the various workhouse boards, and by the guardians from parishes which sent patients to the hospital. He even had to supervise the concert parties put on for the benefit of patients and staff. As if that were not enough, he bore the major load in the training of psychiatric nursing staff. He finished a letter to his mother:

> I have spent all afternoon taking and developing photos of patients, and tomorrow night will be devoted to printing them.

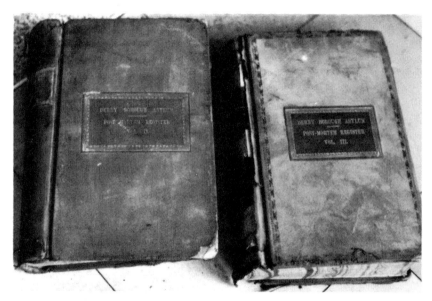

*The autopsy record book, Derby Borough Asylum, 1910-11
(Photograph courtesy of Jean Carr)*

I have to go to lecture to the nurses and attendants this evening, and I must go now and prepare something to say.

Boyd carried out numerous autopsies on patients who were dying in the hospital. In 1911 the causes of death were: phthisis (pulmonary tuberculous)—4, "general paralysis" (syphilitic)—4, heart disease—3, senile exhaustion—5, pneumonia—3, cerebral softening—1, cerebral haemorrhage—1, cerebral tumour—1, epilepsy—1, pernicious anaemia—2, exhaustion of melancholia—2, exhaustion of mania—1, ulcerative colitis—2, locomotor ataxia (syphilitic)—1, cancer of stomach—2, abscess of liver—1, chronic nephritis—1, gastroenteritis—1, pelvic cellulitis—1, tuberculous arthritis—1, gastric ulcer—1. They were the usual causes before the conquest of infectious disease. In the same year at the Derby County Asylum 21 percent of patients died of general paralysis of the insane, as one variety of syphilis affecting the brain was called, and 15.3 percent with phthisis; and epidemic dysentery took its toll.

Boyd's autopsy reports have survived in a heavy leather-bound book. They were the typical brief reports seen in non-teaching hospitals at that time; there was no microscopic examination. There is nothing to suggest in the texts that these apprentice efforts came from the pen of one who would be a master.

During this period he carried out the work on which he based his MD thesis. Many Edinburgh graduates proceeded to the higher degree of MD. The ordinance demanded one year's attendance in wards and scientific work, and an examination in clinical medicine, with a written report and commentary on three medical cases. The thesis had to incorporate either the results of original work, or a full digest and critical exposition of material previously published by others.

Boyd's thesis was titled "On the Cerebrospinal Fluid in Certain Forms of Nervous and Mental Disease". In it he analyzed the changes in the cerebrospinal fluid in a variety of organic brain diseases and psychiatric illnesses. The organism of syphilis, *treponema pallidum*, had recently been incriminated as one of the commonest causes of dementia. The Wasserman serological reaction had been devised as an empirical but effective test for the presence of continued infection; and in 1910 the arsenic compound Salvarsan had been introduced as the first effective treatment for syphilis. It was realized that the control of neurosyphilis demanded that cerebrospinal fluid must be examined repeatedly until it was serolog-

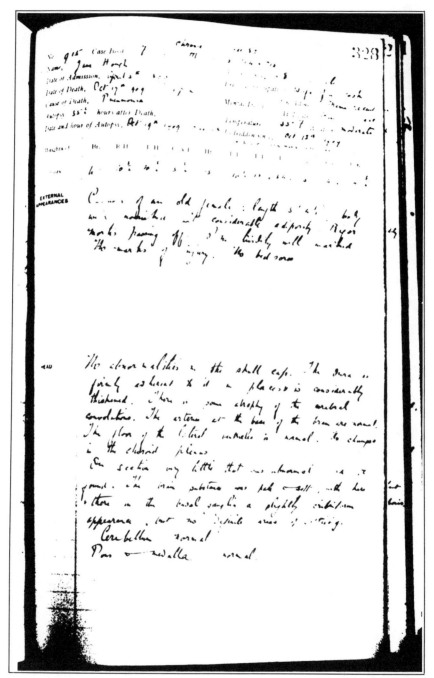

Boyd's first autopsy report (Photograph courtesy of Jean Carr)

CHEST. Ribs on examination found free from recent or old injury. In each pleural sac there was about 10 g of blood stained fluid. The right lung was attached to the parietes by some recent easily broken down adhesions. The apex of the left lung was bound down by extremely strong adhesions which could only be broken down with great difficulty.
Lungs. Both were deeply congested. Interior contains emphysema. Upper lobe of right lung was partially consolidated in a state of "red hepatization". Bronchi showed signs of chronic bronchitis & contained a good deal of mucous fluid.
Heart. No pericardial effusion. Heart muscle not atrophied. Valves are healthy. Mitral orifice admits 2, aortic increased 3 fingers. Aorta shows patches of atheroma.

ABDOMEN. No ascitic fluid. Bowels considerably distended with gas & bound together very firmly so that the various coils could only be separated with the greatest difficulty. Liver was firm & on section showed chronic venous congestion. Gall bladder empty. No gall stones.
Spleen deeply congested, very soft & pliable.
Kidneys. Size was a little less than normal. Capsule stripped easily except in one or two places. No cysts. On section the cortex was found to be rather atrophied. Pyramids normal.
Urinary Bladder contained 2 or 3 oz of urine.
Uterus & appendages normal.

W. Boyd.

Boyd's first autopsy report (contd.)

Rowditch
Derby
12. vii. 10.

My dearest Mother

I have nothing to tell you, & so will write down a prayer I came across to-day. I think it is the finest that I know.

A Prayer for the Day.
O God, give me courage to live another day. Let me not turn coward before its difficulties, or prove recreant to its duties. Let me not lose faith in my fellowmen. Keep me sweet & sound at heart spite of ingratitude, treachery, or meanness. Preserve me, O God, from minding little things, or giving them. Tell me to keep my heart clean, and to live so honestly & fearlessly that no outward thing can dishearten me, or take away

A letter from Boyd to his mother

A letter from Boyd to his mother (contd.)

ically negative. Boyd's thesis contained the results of examination of the cerebrospinal fluid in a wide variety of mental hospital patients.

The thesis revealed no fundamental new discovery, but it was a painstaking and topical work. He still had friends in Edinburgh, and in 1911 graduated MD with honours and a gold medal. The only other honours graduate that year was Kinnier Wilson, who obtained his success and fame with the first description in 1912 of what we now call Wilson's Disease, a genetically determined disorder of copper metabolism affecting the brain and liver.

About this time he became a Member of the Royal College of Physicians of Edinburgh and obtained its Diploma in Psychiatry. As if that were not enough to satisfy his aspirations and pave the way for his future career, he obtained the Diploma in Psychiatry of the Royal Medico-Psychological Association, winning its Gaskell Gold Medal. He was now a formidably qualified young doctor.

The Strong Deliverer

We know little about Boyd's private life in those days. He kept up his student friendship with Alexander Gibson and was still a keen hill-walker and climber — during the period 1909-1911 his hiking diary records walks in Skye and Arran with Gibson.

He wrote regularly to his mother, whose brood was now scattered, and he was still in a conventional sense devout. "I have nothing to tell you, and so will write you a prayer I came across today. O God, give me the courage to live another day. . . . In the name of the strong deliverer. Amen." His Commonplace Book too had quotations of a religious flavour, but we do not know whether he attended the Presbyterian Church in Derby.

He had a liking for Kipling's verse and, probably like many young men of the time, the respect for Empire and the Pax Britannica it extolled. "Iron, cold iron, is the master of them all," he quoted in another letter to his mother; and about this time he joined the Territorial Army.

On the Move Again

Young doctors change jobs for reasons of income and training. In the Annual Report for Winwick Hospital, Warrington, a Lancashire County Asylum, the Medical Superintendent, Dr. Alexander Simpson, was looking for a pathologist to add to his staff of six assistant medical officers.

Boyd was appointed in October 1912, but stayed only till about May 1913. The records show that he actually received only half of his salary of £200.

The report of the scientific investigations for 1912 of Winwick Asylum states:

> The cerebrospinal fluid has been examined in a large number of cases, and the examination has been found to be of great value in diagnosing cases of general paralysis. . . .
>
> Dr. Boyd has carried out vaccine treatment for various conditions, inflammatory skin affections in particular, upon several patients and members of staff, with satisfactory results.
>
> Dr. Boyd has been investigating disturbances of the sympathetic nervous system in mental disorder, more especially in cases of melancholia, two of the chief methods being employed being the administration of Pilocarpine and Adrenalin. Hitherto this subject has received but scant attention, and promising results have been obtained. . . .
>
> WILLIAM BOYD, Pathologist.

The report reveals a man who did not hide his light under a bushel but who knew well how to make what he was doing appear significant, a talent not uncommon in academic medicine, and necessary for those who wish to make any way in it. But it also indicates an aggressive, enquiring, forward-looking mind.

He did not stay long at Winwick and in 1913 was appointed pathologist to Wolverhampton Royal Infirmary. He had already spent some time working for Dr. Carnegie Dickson in bacteriology the previous summer in Edinburgh. Now both Dickson and his former teacher in Edinburgh, Beattie (by then Professor of Pathology and Bacteriology in the University of Liverpool), provided him in early February with warm testimonials indicating that he was trained and committed to a career as a pathologist. He was now taking up a post which involved full-time laboratory investigation of disease. A pathologist had worked in the Infirmary since the end of the previous century under makeshift conditions. Part of the attraction for Boyd must have been the new laboratory, opened by Sir Clifford Allbutt in January 1914. The science of pathology com-

Please come!

prised tissue pathology (histopathology, the microscopic examination of tissues removed surgically), the conduct of autopsies, bacteriology (the characterization of organisms causing disease), and clinical biochemistry (the chemical examination of body fluids). Boyd would have been responsible for all of these. The individual disciplines had not yet expanded to the point where subspecialization was essential. That would develop later during his career. It was a mark of his extraordinary mind that sixty years after his first appointment, he could still write a student textbook which found widespread acceptance, and which covered most of the pathology medical students needed to know.

As at Winwick, his sojourn at Wolverhampton did not last long and left no mark on the hospital pathology department. Gibson wrote to him from Winnipeg suggesting that he apply there, but the guns of August were firing. As he had already joined a Territorial Army Unit, soon after the outbreak of war, on 6 August 1914, he was called to the colours. The minutes of the hospital management committee record that on 25 August 1914, Boyd informed the committee that he had been appointed "Professor of Pathology in the University of Winnipeg [sic]".

Chapter 5

The Nightingale and the Guns — Ypres

THE NEXT phase of Boyd's life was separate, distinct, and deeply and permanently affected him. It is described in his first book, *With a Field Ambulance at Ypres*. The book stands as a portent of the great medical writer to come and as a vivid account of what we have almost forgotten, the horror of "conventional" war. It is dedicated "To the dear memory of my mother", recalling childhood in a manse in far windswept Portsoy on the Moray Firth.

It derives from a series of letters written to his mother, and is described by the author as "not a book, but a diary, written in the kitchens of French farmhouses, in muddy dugouts and other unromantic places, written usually within twenty-four hours of the events described." It is a record of facts, experiences and emotions, "before the facts had become tinged with fiction, the experiences had lost their original sharpness, and the emotions had been erased by the moving finger of time." He prepared it for publication in Winnipeg in August 1916.

He sailed from England early in 1915 (date unstated) and headed "Up to the Firing Line" as a Captain with the 3rd Field Ambulance Unit, attached to the 46th Division of Imperial Forces. They crossed the Channel in the dark with an escort of destroyers from an unnamed port to an unnamed port. "Searchlight after searchlight came into view, sweep-

WITH A FIELD AMBULANCE AT YPRES

BEING LETTERS WRITTEN
MARCH 7—AUGUST 15, 1915

BY

William Boyd

PROFESSOR OF PATHOLOGY, UNIVERSITY OF MANITOBA

ILLUSTRATED

TORONTO
THE MUSSON BOOK COMPANY
LIMITED

The harbinger; — Boyd's first book

ing to and fro upon the face of the waters and lighting up the channel like a vast ballroom." In the dark they nearly ran down a collier from which came the hail, "What ship is that, and where the hell are you going?" They disembarked to spend the first night with the men squeezed into a shed near the quay and the officers on the cobbles outside. Next day they entrained, eight horses and thirty men to a truck, with the officers in first- or second-class carriages.

They detrained at Cassel and marched through the countryside where the first signs of war appeared: "Here and there were little wayside graves bearing the names of English officers."

On the 12th of March he writes, "behind Neuve Chapelle . . . wonderfully interesting day. I had to ride into the little town which is at present the Divisional Headquarters of the Canadians." In the town square he saw the pageantry of war, French soldiers on guard in their red and blue, crestfallen German prisoners-of-war straggling past and a magnificent procession of British lancers still mounted on horses. But reality exploded in a dressing station, a school whose every floor was packed with wounded lying on stretchers on the floor. "It was literally almost impossible to put your foot down without treading on a wounded man." Many men had lain with open wounds in a ploughed field for forty-eight hours.

> One puir Scotch laddie, whose bowels were hanging outside his abdomen, told me that he came from Fife. It was quite like a message from home to hear the broad kindly Scot's tongue again. "I've an awfu' sair belly, doctor."

Boyd had the resilience of youth. As he rode back to his billet he noticed the blackthorn was already beginning to show white — the first touch of spring in a bleak land. The beauty of a bright morning would recall Borrowdale, Land's End, Loch Longside, Lake Louise and Mount Sir Donald. (These last two indicate that the text must have been edited after he had moved to Winnipeg; the Scot soon learned to live in the Twa Countries.)

His mind was still steeped in English literature; he read the *Private Papers of Henry Rycroft*, carried a copy of selections from Browning and quoted Shakespeare, Swinburne and Bright. His phrases call to mind his manse upbringing and Holy Scripture.

He sees afresh; a column on the march is like an immense tinker's encampment on the move. Necessities denied become luxuries. "You need to be really dirty for a few weeks before you can understand anything of the delight of being clean." He does not overlook the pleasures of army life, such as visits by the travelling variety troupe of the "Follies" to entertain the troops at rest behind the front.

His initiation into the fear of death came as a shock. Bullets singing past in the dark aroused "a curious sinking sensation in my epigastric region, and an intense longing to become like the mathematical point which, as Euclid assures us, has position but no magnitude."

The daily round at first consisted of collecting casualties from regimental aid posts in deserted houses, but he records later that he saw in an infectious disease hospital at Bailleul, near Neuve Eglise, measles, mumps, scarlet fever, diphtheria, typhoid, cerebrospinal fever and anthrax, proving the identity of the last by microscopical examination. He was silent on the scourge of gonorrhea and syphilis, a major cause of depletion in the army's strength. Perhaps, for a lay readership, he felt it indelicate to draw attention to a disease which, in those days, was not suitable for public discussion and which would cast disgrace upon men who had volunteered to risk their lives.

He had a "great day with the artillery", and remembered the meshwork of telephone lines across the country, footballers standing stock still at the warning whistle of an aeroplane overhead lest their movement give a clue to the presence of the artillery battery and the dugouts, "tiny chambers, varying from three to four feet in height, roofed with stout timbers, on top of which is a layer of sandbags, with turf sods covering all. In many cases ivy was trained over the roof. Cowslips and violets were planted at the door." At that time sod huts were not rare dwellings either in Manitoba or the Hebrides. Characteristically, the experience of being bombed by a Zeppelin evokes only passing mention. The beauty of the little white puffs of shrapnel bursting around a plane in a cloudless blue sky is noted and relished. In the middle of it all, administrators played their usual games; a telephone message read, "Please send me a return at once of the numbers of great coats in your brigade."

The horror of battle is omnipresent. "Confused fighting in the fields, men simply going for one another with the bayonet or clubbed rifle by the light of the bursting shells, no man knowing where his fellows were or where he was himself." He can sympathize with the enemy, target

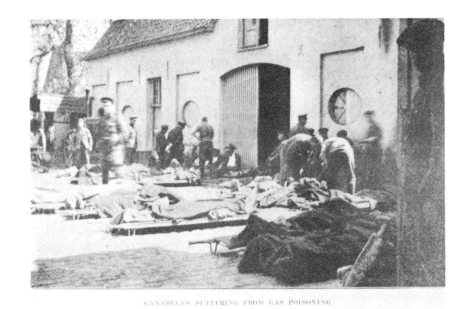

War in Flanders — Canadian casualties of the first gas attack

for the shells from his own side, yet the patriotism of the time stands forth. "It was Canadian versus German, and you can guess which was the better side in a contest of that nature." After nine hours in a dressing station, "all the talk about the glory and glamour of war is apt to stick in one's throat. I am too tired to write any more."

He was among the first to see casualties of gas warfare. On 28 April 1915 he wrote, "There is only one word in the mouth of everyone today — gas." The picture of a casualty clearing station is burned onto the page. "The hospital is built around a great courtyard, and in the courtyard were 200 men on stretchers. Some were lying in a state of stupor, the flies buzzing around their faces; some were sitting up gasping for breath, with hands and faces of a deep dusky hue, evidently in the greatest distress; over the countenance of others the pallid hues of death were beginning to creep, whilst a few had fallen back and with gurglings in the throat were passing away into the undiscovered country. They were the first gas cases from Ypres and Hill 60." The future professor of pathology investigated the serum of severely gassed soldiers in an attempt to find out the nature of the gas, without success.

It was a varied life full of grisly preferences, of shellfire to rifle bullets — "they frighten you more, but do not make you feel so remarkably uncomfortable." Those who rode at night by the light of the starshells, to the rattle of rifle fire, the stutter of machine guns and the sound of howitzers, ran the risks of riding into a telephone wire, having the horse put its foot into a shell hole or being shot in the back by a spy.

One night (he records on 13 May 1915) he walked up a hill with a friend and emerged from the undergrowth onto the hilltop. "The scene that met our eyes was so solemn, so awe-inspiring that all conversation between us ceased. For at our feet lay Ypres burning furiously . . . as we sat, the stillness of the night was broken by the song of birds, faint and hesitating at first, but gradually gathering volume, till the whole air was throbbing with the melody. It was a nightingale singing in the wood below. The whole town was glowing like the mouth of hell . . . at our distance no sound broke the awesome stillness — only the song of the nightingale and the booming of the guns."

He wrote again of a second visit to Ypres (20 May 1915) and quoted, "The cormorant and the bittern shall possess it, the owl also and the raven shall inhabit it, for he hath stretched out upon it the line of confusion, and the stones of emptiness." Yet the darkness did not entirely

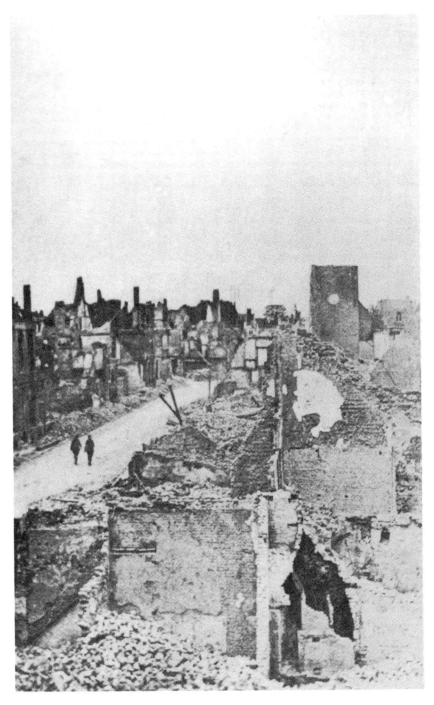

The City of the Dead — the ruins of Ypres

possess him; the nearby Divisional Headquarters, a château, was "like the Backs at Cambridge".

His experience was sometimes gruesome. Like many another he found his way by the dead horse near the Menin Gate; like many another he stumbled over a man with a shattered head and a beating heart, put on a No. 1 field dressing as a token gesture, and passed by; like many another he was arrested as a spy in a dark wood on the Ypres salient. Unlike many, Boyd lived to tell the tale.

Comedy bubbles through as an essential antidote to the heartbreaks. At a dinner party in a dugout, the guests all wore gas goggles, while the gas shells burst down the field. "Silent Sue", they called a large German howitzer. Silent Sue is unheard, "merely arrives and that is the end of the matter. The nature of that end depends entirely on whether or not you happen to be on the spot to receive her."

Military medicine was unprepared for the Great War, for the carnage wrought by the machine gun and by massed concentrations of artillery. There was no precedent for the numbers of wounded who needed emergency surgery, nor for the extensive contamination of wounds by the *clostridium* of gas gangrene. The sanitary conditions experienced by millions of men living and dying for long periods in trenches devoid of sanitation were unique; and there was no precedent for the psychiatric casualties. "Shell-shock" still implied cowardice, rather than pointing to the conclusion that all men must break; the question was not whether, but when.

On 15 July 1915, Boyd recorded the end of his days in the Ypres salient. The University of Manitoba had been requesting his release; he was probably released ultimately because of his commitment to the young Canadian university. He recalls living in one of a row of dugouts when the order came through, and remembers a friend, an athlete, one of those who "make sunshine in the world. A shell burst. And so that is the end of it all."

Boyd, a man who thought that the start of a barrage was like the beginning of Beethoven's Symphony in C Minor, could write on 15 August 1915: "Tomorrow I leave France. . . . All pleasure depends on contrast. The contrasts of war provide an intensity of pleasure which only those who have experienced it can realise." The small, little-known book shows that his pen was tempered at Ypres.

Chapter 6

Prairie Professor

Alec Gibson wrote to Boyd from Winnipeg in June 1914, to tell him that a suitable candidate for the chair of pathology was being sought. "I could help a lot here," he said. By August, Boyd had informed his employers at Wolverhampton that he was going to Winnipeg, but the war intervened, and it was not till late 1915 that he sailed across the Atlantic, a risky passage with German submarines on the prowl.

Winnipeg, Frigid City
For the many people climbing down the steps of the train on a November day in 1915, Winnipeg would have been somewhat of a shock. It was not Edinburgh, nor Derby, but to a young man whose experience of life had included the barren winters of Banffshire and the mud of Flanders it could not have been all that bad. He had expected worse and had heavy hobnail boots ready for the Canadian wilderness. He recollected many years later "clumping hobnails and all across the marble floor of the Fort Garry Hotel, while the orchestra played softly for the tea dance."

There is a good story, probably apocryphal, that his friend Gibson had bribed the guard on the train to Winnipeg to put him off at a halt in the middle of nowhere in the Canadian Shield east of Winnipeg; he

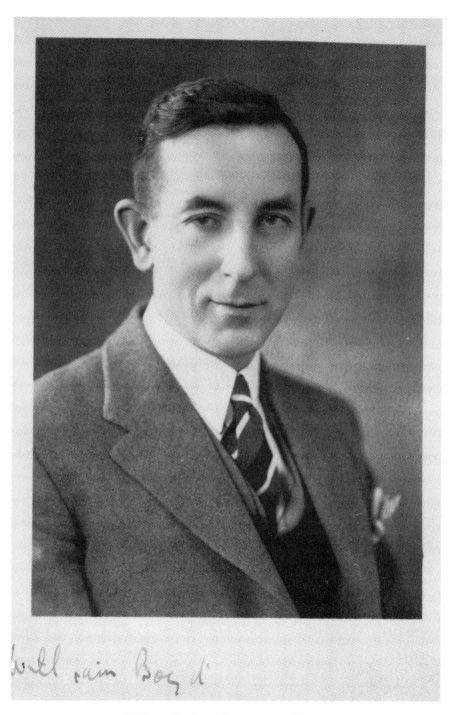

William Boyd — the young professor

was dumped with his baggage on an empty platform in the dark. After a cold quarter of an hour, Alexander Gibson jumped from behind a bush, filled him with Scotch from his hip flask, and took him off to a nearby cottage.

In 1915 Winnipeg was still a young city. It had grown slowly at the Forks of the Red and Assiniboine rivers after the foundation of the Red River Colony in 1812. The initial settlers had been the Kildonan Scots and migrants from Ontario. St. Boniface across the river was settled by Francophones. However, after 1870 Manitoba had become a province, and the western Canadian prairies were opened up mostly by settlers from Eastern Europe.

The city was cold and isolated but had the beginnings of style, nurtured by a period of great commercial prosperity. This was abruptly halted in 1913 when the opening of the Panama Canal led to exports by-passing cross-country shipment. The unfinished exteriors of several grandiose Winnipeg buildings still testify to its misfortune. The city flourished on the profits of the grain trade and of a mixed group of industries. It was linked to the rest of the world by the railway; road access in 1915 was still incomplete. The new Legislative building was inaugurated in 1920 and gave off a whiff of financial scandal from the disclosure of peculation by contractors. The population was 136,000 in 1911, and 160,000 in 1916. The growth slowed down after 1929, but the population reached 216,000 in 1936. The rich and successful lived in large ornate mansions and gathered in the Manitoba Club. The upper and middle classes had a good life which briefly recreated that of Edwardian England, at least until the "Proud Tower" (European civilization as it was before World War I) collapsed in 1914. Tennis parties, boating and canoeing were usual recreations, while some of the rich entertained themselves with fox hunting.

Boyd was paid $4000 per annum at a time when a ticket to the movies cost 15 cents, and a cleaning woman charged 20 cents an hour.

Recent eastern European immigrants lived in great poverty in the North End, looked down upon by the Anglo-Canadian establishment. There was great social polarization, accompanied by frequent labour unrest. The poor lived very poorly indeed in shanty towns often lacking clean water and adequate sanitation. Epidemics of typhoid, smallpox, scarlet fever and diphtheria filled the graveyards, particularly in the spring. The Winnipeg red light district was a byword. Police wearing helmets, like London bobbies, walked the beat and enforced the law with truncheons. Peace, order and good government were further upheld when necessary by the Royal North West Mounted Police.

In 1918 the Spanish influenza epidemic caused many deaths, and public concern rose to the point of panic. Public meetings were banned for seven weeks in Winnipeg, and the medical school was temporarily closed. There was work for a young pathologist.

As Boyd walked for the first time down the wide main streets, he saw electric streetcars and a few automobiles, but horses were more obvious; and, until the 1920s, oxen still plodded down the road as they dragged their creaking carts behind them. Cars parked next to hitching posts. The city was still subject to spring floods, sometimes very severe. From the 3rd of April to the 2nd of May in 1916, basements were flooded over wide areas of the city, and there was no gas or electricity in one hospital for two weeks.

In late 1915 the predominant emotion in Winnipeg was patriotism, and the main topic of thought and conversation the War. Money was raised and comforts, usually knitted, were prepared for soldiers. The slaughter in Flanders left gaps in many households as frenzied hatred, directed at the enemy, gathered momentum. At first, Boyd was active in lecturing to public audiences all over Western Canada and in Grand Forks, North Dakota, on his war experiences, in tones which show that he clearly (and understandably) shared in the war hysteria of the time. He talked of the beastly Boche, or Hun, and gave accounts, which may well have been true, of war atrocities. His attitude later mellowed to an elegiac sadness.

Winnipeg was a city studded with churches. The puritan Presbyterian Church, in one of whose manses Boyd was to find his future wife, was strong, attracting twenty-two percent of churchgoers. The demon drink was much hated, and in 1916 a form of prohibition existed, mitigated in 1923 by a provincial monopoly liquor control board. There were civilized entertainments — fourteen theatres in 1920 ranging from classical repertory and visiting companies, to vaudeville, circus and, increasingly in the 1920s, cinema. By 1930 most comfortably off families had a radio and a phonograph.

The Winnipeg General Strike of 1919 was a symptom of social division, and created much rancour; for four years or so afterwards industrial depression persisted. No hint exists in Boyd's letters to suggest that he was particularly concerned about the social conditions around him; he was well paid.

The Manitoba Medical College

Boyd was appointed to the Manitoba Medical College, which was not yet in name the Faculty of Medicine of the University of Manitoba. The medical school was young and inadequately housed, the faculty strained by the War. A new pathology building was nearly ten years in the future. Boyd had been appointed by what would now be called influence. To understand the story, it is necessary to understand a little of the development of the Manitoba Medical College.

The Manitoba Medical College, founded in 1883, had been at first a very small enterprise, part of the community's attempt to raise health standards. It grew and improved over the next twenty-five years. The dominant administrative figure over the first seventeen years of the new century was Henry Havelock Chown, a skilful surgeon who was appointed Dean in 1900. Throughout his period of office there was a struggle to establish basic science, good hospital care and specialist medicine, and to control tuberculosis and other infectious diseases. The burgeoning science of bacteriology was fundamental in the plan, advocated and led by Dr. Gordon Bell.

The medical school was inspected in 1909 by the Flexner Commission which was appraising the standard of medical schools across North America. The report noted the high standard of medical practice in the Winnipeg General Hospital, but placed the Manitoba Medical College in the second class of medical schools because it lacked, in particular, proper laboratory and teaching space. The stigma of being a second-class educational establishment was the stimulus for reform. The Dean, who was left in no doubt that he should acquire some professional pre-clinical teachers, had taken his postgraduate surgical diploma in Edinburgh, the pre-eminent medical centre in the British Empire. After one unsuccessful recruiting attempt, Chown knew where to turn.

"What Pull Can Do"

Alexander Gibson, Boyd's classmate, had graduated in 1908 at Edinburgh, the brightest student by far of his day. He had recently qualified as a Fellow of the Royal College of Surgeons. Chown offered him the Chair of Anatomy and reported by telegram to the Faculty of Medicine: "Have got Gibson, able, agreeable."

Thus was anatomy looked after; but more faculty appointments were needed. At a time when the links with Scotland were much stronger than they are now it was natural to look in the same direction. In 1913, the University was looking for a Professor of Pathology to put into effect some of the reforms recommended in the Flexner Report. In May 1913, the faculty resolved that "the Registrar be instructed to write the University requesting that a Professor of Pathology be appointed at the earliest possible date, said Professor to be paid by the University." Alexander Gibson had a crony with whom he had walked the Cuillin and the hills of Arran. So he wrote to William Boyd, then Pathologist to Wolverhampton Royal Infirmary, on 9 June 1914.

> My dear Will, I received your welcome letter about two weeks ago, and now hasten to reply to it. First of all, the Dean came to me yesterday, and asked if I knew anyone who would do for the post of first Professor of Pathology, in this University. I said I did, and asked the terms. Subjects to be taught — Pathology and Histology. Remuneration: Pathology $3,000; Histology $1,000 — Total $4,000. Put that under your tongue. The authorities are writing to Osler at Oxford and Sims Woodhead at Cambridge, but I could help a whole lot here, I think.
>
> If you could see the sunshine we get here, it would almost persuade you. If you get the job, I'll introduce you to a keen mountaineering man who goes to the Rockies every July. Man, it would be fine for us to be together again.

The salary offered was princely compared with what Boyd was being paid at Wolverhampton — £200 sterling a year.

Two months later the Dean reported progress in the matter of securing a Professor of Pathology, and on 11 September 1914, he announced that Dr. William Boyd had been appointed by the University as Professor of Pathology. A request was received by the War Office in London that Boyd be allowed three months leave of absence, later to be extended to a year. Boyd was at the time committed to service in the Army Medical Corps in France and did not arrive in Winnipeg until November 1915, more than a year after his official appointment.

The hospital and medical school to which Boyd came already had some established standards in pathology, although it was still a young subject. Since 1897 Dr. Gordon Bell had been Provincial Bacteriologist and first Professor of Pathology, Bacteriology and Histology. Because of the ravages of infectious disease, his first priority had been to develop a bacteriology service. In 1907, Dr. Sidney J.S. Pierce was appointed as his assistant. He had graduated three years previously from the Manitoba Medical School and had had a year's training with Bell himself, and two years at the Mayo Clinic at Rochester, Minnesota. For the next seven years, until Boyd's appointment, he was largely responsible for the collection and preparation of teaching material, and for lecturing and examining in Pathology with Professor Bell.

Ructions
Boyd was appointed over the head of Pierce, the local candidate. Boyd himself had less actual experience as a pathologist, but this was offset by his shining academic qualifications — MD by thesis with honours from Edinburgh University, Membership of the Royal College of Physicians of Edinburgh and a gold medal in psychiatry.

Boyd was to write much later: "Although I had never in my life given a lecture in Pathology (or any other subject) or even demonstrated to one student, I got the job. Which shows what pull can do — if you have the right man pulling the wire." He also admitted that he spent much of his time crossing the Atlantic preparing 100 lectures on pathology, from Mallory's newly published *Principles of Pathologic Histology*. "Of course, I knew very little pathology, but then the boys knew nothing. I managed to keep one day ahead of them by reading up at night."

There were, as might have been expected, ructions in the Winnipeg General Hospital and the Faculty of Medicine. Dr. Pierce resigned on 8 October 1915, but was persuaded by a committee appointed by the Dean to withdraw his resignation. Dean Chown resigned his connection with the Winnipeg General Hospital, and thus, as he explained to the Faculty on 11 November 1915, could no longer be a member of the Faculty nor Dean of the College. Another committee was appointed which reported back to Faculty on 10 December 1915 that "Dr. Chown's resignation from the Hospital had been withdrawn, and consequently the Medical College work would go on as usual." The hullaballoo Boyd walked into must have seemed a storm in a teacup after the Western Front.

The relationship between Hospital and University Pathology Department was to be further defined by a committee consisting of Chown, Prowse (the next Dean, and a potent figure in the Medical School) and Boyd. The Dean and the University had won, and pathology in the Manitoba Medical School and Winnipeg General Hospital was to be controlled by Boyd for twenty years.

The very effective University takeover of pathology at the Winnipeg General was recorded in a memo dated 10 March 1916: "The pathological work of the Hospital and the College to be united under one head and the work to be carried on in the College." The College was to furnish space and equipment except for what it took over from the Hospital. The College was to control appointments, except that the Hospital would have a say in what the intern staff was to do. The Hospital was to pay the College salaries and board for two interns.

Pierce accepted an appointment as Associate Professor of Pathology but left after two years to take charge of laboratories in Brandon. Dr. Long, who had been the bacteriologist, left more immediately for a job in Minnesota. Boyd now had a clear field.

The loss of staff members who were there when Boyd was appointed had some temporary effect. Two laboratory physicians left and the teaching of clinical pathology to students and interns stopped for a time. Only eighteen autopsies were conducted that year as opposed to fifty-eight in 1909. Boyd did not yet have the tact to handle a difficult administrative situation; at that time Professor, particularly in Scotland whence Boyd came, was spelt with a very large P, and implied divinity.

In March 1917, the laboratories of the General Hospital were moved to a three-storey brick-and-stone building which had been built in 1894 and had formerly been the nurses' residence for an isolation hospital. Boyd's office and the surgical pathology laboratory were situated on the first floor. Half the second floor was occupied by the histology, microbiology and urinalysis laboratories. The other half became the biochemistry laboratory the following year. Half the third floor consisted of sleeping quarters for the Chinese cooks at the Hospital. The building was connected by tunnel with the Medical School, the power house and the hospital. Boyd was to work in these rather makeshift quarters until the new Pathology Building was opened in 1924. It provided ampler quarters, particularly space to develop an extensive Pathological Museum.

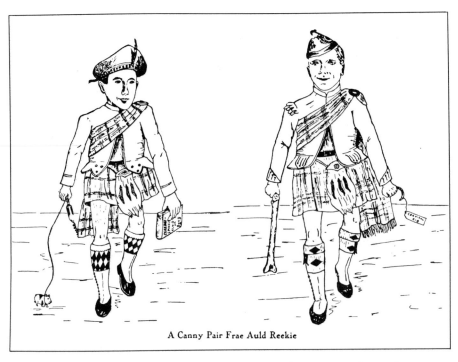

The Two Jocks — William Boyd and J.C.B. Grant — as the students saw them

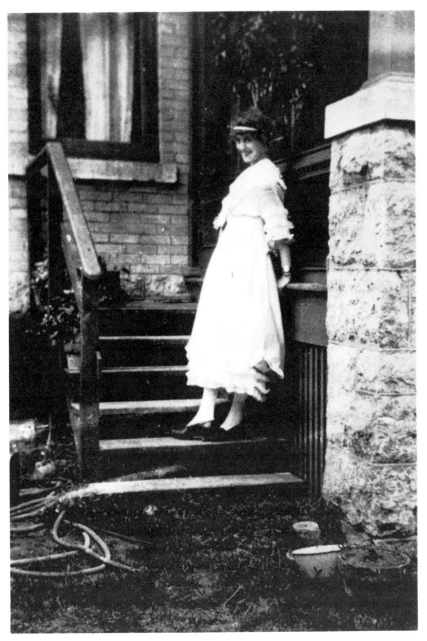

Days in Arcady — Enid

The College and the University
In 1919 the College became the Faculty of Medicine of the University of Manitoba. It was still a small institution; Medical Faculty Council met on occasion in the home of the Dean. The small Faculty consisted largely of local men, with an infusion of Scots: thus in 1919 Grant was Professor of Anatomy, Swale Vincent was Professor of Physiology, Gordon Bell was Professor of Bacteriology. They were able men who for the most part had made or would make national reputations; but their style was a far cry from the knighted and haughty professoriate of the University of Edinburgh. Edinburgh Medical School had seen the discovery of chloroform anaesthesia and the early days of antiseptic surgery before the Manitoba Medical College opened.

The private practice of medicine was still very important in Winnipeg in 1919; there were no full-time clinical professors in the faculty. Clinical professors made their livelihood from private fees. There was a wrangle in Medical Faculty Council on 22 November 1922 when Dr. Daniel Nicholson wanted to open a private laboratory for the Medical Arts Building where the clinical teaching staff saw their patients in private offices. Boyd is not recorded as having strong views on this matter. He had a growing but never dominant influence and, as late as 25 July 1930, was to complain that he had been ill used in the matter of the dismissal of a technologist.

Dean Prowse had also done his postgraduate training in Edinburgh and favoured Scottish medical patterns. In many areas of life, academic and otherwise, the influence of the "old country" and of things British remained strong. The men who dominated the Manitoba Medical School in the 1920s, Canadian and British, were deeply marked by their experiences in the trenches. Boyd's war service gave him significant local standing.

Days in Arcady. Private life.
We know a fair bit about Boyd's life in Winnipeg from faculty minutes and from his correspondence with his fiancée, Enid, the daughter of David Christie, the minister of Westminster Presbyterian Church, to whom Boyd had presented a letter of introduction on his arrival. Churches were more natural centres of social life than they are now, and Boyd had grown up in a Church background. While in his later years his religious faith faded, the Free Church in which he grew up had imparted a good knowl-

edge of the scriptures. It is evident from his Commonplace Book that his reading was, at least until 1937, deeply serious. It is likely that after World War I he drifted quite quickly away from orthodox Christian beliefs.

The letters to Enid when they were courting are affectionate, but with an undertone of fret and distress. Their disputes were about trivial things, a party missed, a remark misinterpreted as slighting. "You with your craving for excitement would not consider that as having a good time."

They enjoyed simple pleasures, a holiday in Enid's parents lakeside cottage at Matlock, trips to Grand Beach, which advertized itself just after the war as the Bathers' Paradise. Girls' knees could now be seen on the bathing beach, and there was dancing in the Big Pavilion. They went canoeing on Lake of the Woods, where a friend often lent Enid's parents a cottage on an island near Kenora. Boyd wrote, while on a 1917 stay in New York, of the pleasure of shopping in Winnipeg and other mundane pastimes.

It took Boyd years to feel settled in Winnipeg. At first he had a period of professional indecision. He visited New York in 1917 and his correspondence with Enid shows that he was still hankering after his clinical life, perhaps returning to neurology, which included psychiatry. He still thought of returning to Europe. He wished that his medical career could start all over again. He did not enjoy the hassles which were a part of the hospital side of his job. "I think that whatever else I do I should give up the hospital; I only wish that I had never been persuaded into having anything to do with the place." He writes poignantly of his anxiety over friends wounded in France, and of his sorrow over lost friends, Enid's brother, and another "who was one of the finest classical scholars I have known, and who carried a copy of the *Oddyssey* [sic] in Greek with him wherever he went." His sister even asked him in a letter in 1917 whether he was still thinking of returning to the war.

In New York he enjoyed the metropolitan pleasures and worried a little like all young men whether his girlfriend was two-timing him. While he was at the New York Neurological Institute he found a publisher for his book on the cerebrospinal fluid (the book was largely rewritten in Boston and New York during this trip). He had the chance of re-entering clinical medicine through an invitation to stay as senior resident at the Peter Bent Brigham Hospital, an excellent starting spot for academic or consultant practice; but he chose Enid and Winnipeg.

He already enjoyed the sound of his own voice. After describing how

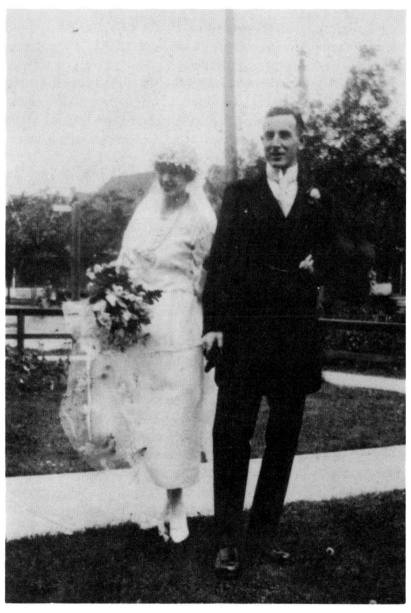

Newly wed

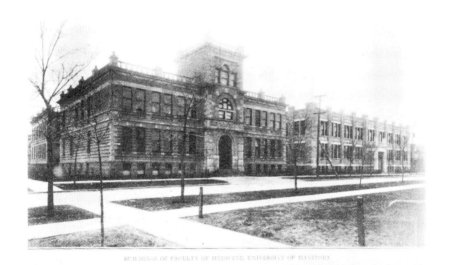

The Manitoba Medical School in the 1920s

on holiday at Thetford, Ontario, at his brother Guy's farm he enjoyed pitching hay and playing with the children, he continued,

> This morning (Sunday, July 23rd 1918) I occupied the pulpit of the Presbyterian church, read the lesson and preached the sermon. There was a joint meeting of the Methodists and Presbyterians, and tonight there is to be another joint service in the Methodist church at which I again officiate. The church was packed to the very back, and I really got in touch with my audience and got carried away. At the end I saw tears running over the faces of the farmers' wives which they furtively mopped up — quite a triumph, eh? I think I must give up medicine for the pulpit: I believe that I really could fill a city church.

At this stage he was still conventionally religious quoting (9 September 1918) Browning: "God's greatness flows around our incompleteness." However, he thinks not of how well he pleased the Deity, but how much he enjoyed the power of having a church full of people hanging on his words. From the comments of many of his later friends a large part of the man was actor. He was usually financially better off than his brothers and he lent or gave them money. "It generally results in my being soft headed enough to part with some of my hoarded gold, with the result that I shall never have enough to marry."

It was a June wedding, Monday, 2 June 1919, and the bride's father married them in Westminster Church, Winnipeg. "The bride, daintily attired in white silk with a French hand-embroidered net veil, enwreathed in orange blossoms, carried a shower bouquet of bridal roses and orchids." Alexander Gibson was the best man. The honeymoon was spent "in the south", said the newspaper notice. In fact, Boyd took Enid to Europe, probably to Switzerland, where he climbed the Matterhorn. The joy of a honeymoon was complete only among the mountains.

He lived well in a new, comfortable, middle-class house, 77 Queenston Street, and drove one of the first electric motor cars in Winnipeg. He enjoyed dancing, and with his friend J.C.B. Grant, who arrived in Winnipeg in 1919, took care to learn the latest steps. He liked the new entertainment — the cinema. By 1921, flowers and his flower garden meant a great deal to him. He writes of "a great vase of tulips but only one was a patch on mine". There was a longing for the mountains —

his basement had a climbing frame on the wall, and he went hiking and climbing frequently, usually in the Rockies.

Enid herself was his intellectual peer, a University gold medallist in Greek. Initially she fretted a little over her husband's dedication to his career, and went dancing while Will foregathered of an evening with his students in a café to eat onion sandwiches. But she was soon a good Faculty wife, settled to domesticity and the social round.

By 1921 his marriage had tied him to Winnipeg, where Enid's family was important to her. The modest success of his first medical book pointed his way to the future, and the opening of the new pathology building in 1924 had made him feel an important part of the Medical School.

The Young Professor

Boyd was Professor of Pathology in the University and Chief Pathologist to the Winnipeg General Hospital, described by the Flexner Report as an excellent hospital. In the former capacity he lectured to a class of sixty medical students, taught gross pathology in the autopsy room and microscopic pathology in the laboratory, all in the traditional Edinburgh manner — "a young man with an eager face and a Scottish accent, an excellent lecturer and a perfect gentleman".

In May 1919, Boyd had the chance to appoint, as his own assistant, Dr. Daniel Nicholson, who had graduated in Winnipeg with the Gold Medal in 1919. Nicholson was at first Assistant Pathologist at the General Hospital and then Lecturer in Pathology at the University. Boyd controlled appointments to both hospital and university departments. He notes in his report to the Board of the General Hospital in 1920 that Dr. Daniel Nicholson had undertaken the whole of the autopsy service, and "performed it in so excellent a manner." In 1924 Nicholson became Associate Pathologist at the General Hospital and Associate Professor of Pathology and succeeded Boyd in 1937. Nicholson's successor was Dr. John Lederman, also a pupil and junior colleague of Boyd, so that the Boyd stamp remained on Winnipeg pathology.

He learned early of the advantages of the cultivation of well-known figures in medicine; in a letter from his sister Win, dated 15 July 1917, she notes that he had just visited Rochester and the Mayos. In 1922 James Ewing, the great New York pathologist, visited him in Winnipeg.

In 1924, the new Pathology Building opened. With ample lecture and laboratory space Boyd, by now secure in his specialty and in his place

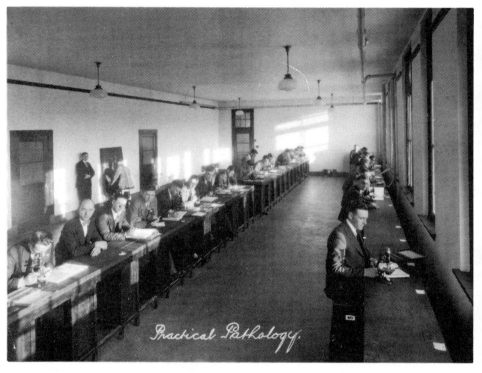

Manitoba medical students in the 1920s — in the pathology laboratory

With the author's comps.
W. Boyd

Reprinted from THE CANADIAN MEDICAL ASSOCIATION JOURNAL,
February, 1920

THE WINNIPEG EPIDEMIC OF ENCEPHALITIS LETHARGICA

BY WILLIAM BOYD, M.D.

Winnipeg

WHETHER to the internist, the neurologist, the pathologist, or the epidemiologist lethargic encephalitis is a disease of absorbing interest. The geographic distribution and general epidemic behaviour of this mysterious disease are baffling to a degree. In distinction to influenza which swept over Europe with express trains, crossing the Atlantic with fast liners, and wandering through Asia with camel caravans, epidemic encephalitis appears now here, now there, descending on the startled community like a bolt from the blue. In this it bears a close resemblance to acute poliomye-

An early paper; this made Boyd's name as a pathologist

in the city, spread his wings and over the succeeding years developed an excellent pathological museum, rich in correlation between clinical history and pathological specimen. Students flocked to it. It became a place where students met and talked about pathology and many other things amongst themselves and with the Professor and his colleagues. The museum took much space, ultimately in 1937 about 7000 square feet. Many years later when fashions in teaching were changing, his successors dismantled it, to Boyd's regret.

In the hospital he performed autopsies and examined pathological tissues removed at surgical operations. He was responsible for the pathological examination of some fluids, notably cerebrospinal fluid. In his correspondence with his fiancée he had described the hospital part of his job as stressful. The House Committee wrote to ask why "Dr. Pierce and I were away at the same time, and when I was coming back to take up work again. I nearly wrote telling them to go to Hell."

He carried out autopsies in coroners' cases to which a fee was attached. Another occasional source of extra income was the collecting of cerebrospinal fluid from a private patient. "Burridge drove me over to Polson Ave., where I extracted $10 and some C.S.F. from one of your Hebrew friends." The snide phrase is typical of the anti-Jewish sentiment of the day. The fee was his to keep.

As the specialty of pathology expanded, Boyd was able to shuck off responsibility for the things which interested him the least. In 1920, A.T. Cameron was appointed Associate Professor of Physiological Chemistry followed shortly by the opening of larger laboratories which allowed the development of the biochemistry service.

The cost of laboratories was still quite low — the expenditures of the Department of Pathology in 1920 give an idea of the scale of things: salaries and wages cost $6,745.48, supplies $557, for a total of $7,302.48. Even allowing for an inflation factor of 100, the figure is far short of the laboratory budget of a comparable hospital in 1991.

It was epidemic time. Hardly had the populace recovered from the influenza pandemic of 1918 when, during the winter of 1919-1920, Winnipeg experienced a major outbreak of encephalitis lethargica ("sleeping sickness"). It was Boyd's big chance and he took it. He published excellent pathological accounts of this and a later epidemic. He wrote in his annual report to the Board of the Hospital for 1920, "It is believed that this is one of the most extensive investigations into the pathology of epidemic encephalitis which has hitherto been undertaken." He had adopted New World magniloquence. But his published work on these epidemics became the basis of his reputation as a pathologist.

In 1920 he stated that he was offered an appointment as Professor of Pathology in the Egyptian Government School of Medicine, and Pathologist to the Kasr-el-Ain Hospital at Cairo. He decided, however, to remain in Winnipeg. It was the first of several such temptations.

As the years went by, Boyd himself did less work in the hospital although he continued in active pathology practice throughout his time in Winnipeg. For example, in 1924, 139 autopsies were carried out, mostly by Dr. Boyd. Boyd's autopsy protocols were brief, without clinical summaries of the cases. The brain was examined only when clinically indicated, and the spinal cord was rarely studied. Histologic examination was often selective or absent rather than routinely inclusive of all body tissues. Sometimes photographic illustrations were included in the reports. A year later, in 1925, 158 autopsies were conducted — less than a third by Boyd, the rest by two residents, Dr. John McEachern, who became an internist, and Dr. Sara Meltzer, who the next year became a member of the staff of the Pathology Department and who worked in the General Hospital till her premature death in 1942. In contrast to Boyd's, her autopsy protocols were detailed, included complete clinical summaries and were often illustrated with photographs.

As is usual, the University Department trained non-academic pathologists for the city, among them men who severally founded large Winnipeg private pathology practices, serving major Winnipeg hospitals.

The Silver Pen
Boyd had always been a scribbler. His habit of writing out quotations taken from his reading in a Commonplace Book stimulated his literary talent, filling his mind with quotable phrases and influencing his style.

His first paper appeared within two years and his MD thesis within three years of his graduation. An account of his experiences in Flanders followed (please see Chapter 5). Its favourable reception in papers in Winnipeg, New York and London must have confirmed his hope that he had a real talent for writing. Shortly after arriving in Winnipeg, during a visit to New York he found a publisher for a short book on the cerebrospinal fluid which was an expansion of his MD thesis. By 1920, he was probably chafing at the routine nature of his duties or at the backwater in which he found himself. Ambition stirred in him and his mind turned to the planning of another book. He used to write in longhand, mostly early in the morning. From about 1922, writing dominated his life.

He first wrote a few papers to prove himself as an academic surgical pathologist, and followed these up by a book for surgeons (*Pathology for the Surgeon*, 1st edition 1925). It was the prescribed textbook for the Winnipeg medical students the next year. By 1925 Boyd must have come to the conclusion that he was good at writing textbooks. He wrote steadily over the next few years: *Pathology of Internal Disease* (1931) and *Textbook of Pathology* (1932) were to make his name.

The Golden Tongue
It soon became evident that Boyd was a natural and outstanding teacher. The quotations in his Commonplace Book in the early 1920s of passages from great orators show that he was becoming preoccupied with the art of public speaking. Although his reputation rested on teaching and on his books rather than on research, there was little change in the undergraduate curriculum in pathology during the twenty years that Boyd was Professor. His great contribution lay not so much in what he taught as in how he taught it. His particular contribution was how he taught the scientific basis of disease as part of human medicine rather than simply morbid anatomy as a dead, circumscribed subject.

His students and technologists saw and heard a young man with an eager face, the smooth manner of a gentleman and a splendid lecturer with a pronounced but not broad Scottish accent. The perfection of his lecturing was enhanced rather than marred by an idiosyncrasy in his speech, an inability to trill the letter "r". He always spoke of "bwonchitis".

He was popular with students and played a part in their life outside the classroom, partly because he came to appreciate and enjoy the many good things about living in Winnipeg. In reply to a toast at a students' dinner in the 1920s he said:

> "When I came to Winnipeg a few years ago, I could not help noticing certain differences between this University and my old school at Edinburgh. I was perhaps most impressed by the decorum of the Western student, his serious view of life. Over in Auld Reekie there were far more hare-brained scapegraces, and they

led some of the unfortunate professors a dog's life. One of our chief occupations in the class of physics was to prepare paper darts which we used to throw at the poor professor as soon as his back was turned when drawing on the board, and when the lights were turned out for a lantern demonstration there were loud noises of osculation calculated to embarrass both the professor and the lady students who occupied the front benches.

"We live in a young land which in itself is a great stimulus, and we live at a time of rebirth and reawakening."

His speeches were full of quotations and lambent with idealism: again and again he exhorted his juniors to be charitable — to avoid the cutting word. "My chief regrets are for the unkind things I have said, and doing things that hurt other people."

Boyd had been hired by Dean Chown to help to raise the Manitoba Medical School to the first rank. On 15 November 1923 the American Medical Association Council on Medical Education and Hospitals wrote to the Dean, "Your medical school has now been entered among our class A medical schools." They had made it. The standard had taken forty years to establish. The three men from Edinburgh (Gibson, Grant and Boyd) had played a significant part in the reforms.

As an organizer of teaching, Boyd was a pragmatic modifier, rather than a fundamental innovator. The pathology curriculum when he arrived was similar to that in most British and Canadian medical schools. Boyd did not greatly change the subject matter, but improved the course by his excellent lecturing, Socratic teaching and development of the pathology museum.

In 1916 general pathology was taught in the second year, consisting of twenty-five lectures and fifty two-hour laboratory classes, a total of 125 hours. Special pathology was taught in third year, with fifty lectures and fifty laboratory sessions for a total of 275 hours over the two years. In addition, Dr. Pierce taught clinical pathology in the laboratory of the General Hospital. A major curriculum review in 1921 left pathology intact. In 1931 a second-year examination in pathology was introduced. By 1935 about the same number of hours were devoted to pathology as in 1915. Throughout Boyd's tenure, students had to attend at least six autopsies.

In addition to lectures, demonstrations, laboratory classes and a class in clinical pathology, third- and fourth-year students attended clinico-pathological conferences every Saturday morning. These were important. At first they were poorly attended by staff clinicians. Boyd complained in 1920, "On the only two occasions when the clinicians have turned up, they have been so late and have taken so little trouble to get up the history of the case that it would really be more satisfactory if one could get the use of a good history." But soon afterwards he withdrew his complaint; the clinicians realized how good the sessions were and began to attend faithfully.

They were right; the man who was to become the greatest pathology teacher of his generation was by his fortieth birthday worthy of attention.

— Chapter 7 —

Halfway

By THE MIDDLE of 1929 William Boyd, at the age of 44, was firmly established nationally and internationally, and almost halfway through what was to be a long life. He had, however, already turned down at least one offer to leave Winnipeg, and no doubt could have found a congenial job elsewhere had he so desired. His position as a prairie professor still satisfied him, enlivened as it was by an ever increasing number of academic forays elsewhere in Canada and the United States. He was still slim, erect and fast moving, with his Scottish accent little affected by his years on the prairie. His initial reputation as war hero was fading as the memory of the war became less keen. But he was an established member of the coterie of ex-servicemen who believed it was their right to control the Medical School and Hospital. He was held in considerable esteem by the physicians and surgeons of the Winnipeg General Hospital. His teaching and his teaching methods were popular.

In the *University of Manitoba Medical Journal* in 1928 there were accounts of the obviously popular Saturday morning conferences "conducted by the Professors of Pathology and Medicine". "I see Dr. Boyd smiling to himself. I think he must have something up his sleeve," a clinical teacher would declare, anticipating the exposure of his wrong diagnosis by Boyd's autopsy revelation.

He was in charge of a small but competent pathology department with capable assistants whom he had appointed. It is probable that in 1915 the standard of teaching in pathology in Winnipeg was significantly lower than in major centres in Great Britain and the United States. By 1937, standards had risen significantly. He played an important though not pre-eminent part in the administration of the College, on curriculum and library committees and the like.

The Dean was a surgeon with whom he got on well. Financially Boyd was comfortably off. He was happily married and settled, though childless. There is some suggestion that he was perturbed that he might carry genes which contributed to his sister's severe psychiatric illness.

He had published three books, all well received, but fame was still ahead of him. He was working hard on the *Pathology of Internal Disease*, to be published in 1931. By now he had sufficient experience in pathology to be credible. The *Textbook of Pathology* (1932) was an immediate success and made his name. Within a year it was a recommended medical student text in a large number of North American and British medical schools. Just before he left for Toronto in 1937, he completed the series with a readable little text for student technologists. These books were all written in Winnipeg, went into repeated editions, were translated into several languages and made their author wealthy. Later on in old age, a survivor of a parotid gland tumour, he wrote on a subject that has fascinated many pathologists — the spontaneous regression of tumours.

The books made his reputation, first in Winnipeg, then, when the *Textbook of Pathology* appeared, round the medical world. Other Canadian academic pathologists were critical, and prescribed other reading for their students. Even the University of Toronto, which was to welcome him as its own a few years later, advised its students to turn to other sources, advice which many students chose to ignore. Colleagues, who may have known more about pathology but could not write readably, could not bring themselves to recommend to their students the writings of an erstwhile psychiatrist turned self-taught pathologist. Nor could they admit that Boyd's influence lay in his power with words, a talent they did not possess.

A Memory Snapshot
Dr. Harry Medovy, one of the great figures of the Manitoba Medical

Faculty in the period 1960-1980 gives a bright memory snapshot of Boyd around this time.

> I spent two summers as a medical student resident in pathology under Dr. Boyd (1926 and 1927). We worked in the old Infectious Disease Building. Boyd was busy writing his textbook of Pathology and he lectured to us from the manuscript. I recall (his junior staff) checking the proofs. Boyd was a superb lecturer — full of phrases that lingered in the mind [e.g.] papilloma of the bladder—like leaves floating in a limpid pool.
>
> I spent the year 1929-30 in Philadelphia doing a residency in paediatrics. I received a note from Dr. Boyd, I think in March 1930, that he was coming down to Philadelphia to see about getting a publisher for his textbook. I recall that he had been encouraged by Saunders and Co. to submit his manuscript. He was crest-fallen and shattered when Saunders informed him that McCallum's Textbook was one of their most successful medical textbooks (McCallum was Professor of Pathology in Johns Hopkins Medical School) and that therefore they could not handle two large textbooks of Pathology. They suggested that he should see Lea & Febiger across the road. That afternoon I picked up two tickets for Wagner's "Parsifal" — the Metropolitan Opera production conducted by Tullio Serafin. The opera lasted five hours and we were both exhausted by the experience, although we enjoyed it very much. The next morning, Boyd saw Lea & Febiger who undertook publication. The rest is history. It turned out to be one of the best-selling medical textbooks ever published.
>
> I remember his interest in mountain climbing, and a very dramatic evening lecture on his experiences as a mountain climber in Switzerland. He went into great detail about equipment and how he practised climbing on the wall of his basement.
>
> Boyd loved classical music — he had a sizeable collection of records — the first to get a complete set of all the Beethoven 32 sonatas recorded by Artur Schnabel. He played some of them for us at his home, and kept us informed about concerts he had been to on one of his lecture tours.

Boyd had one of the few electric automobiles in the city. I recall a ride in it — very quiet and very slow. I believe it was quite expensive and a real status symbol.

He was primarily an educator — a "bridge man". He did little research, but he could make a complex area come to life in vivid prose and he had a great memory for detail.

Boyd chose to live on the plains, or they chose him; but the image of the mountains shone in his soul, and he made the pilgrimage to the Rockies as often as he could, often with Enid, and often with colleagues. He recorded his exaltation of high places in articles in the *Winnipeg Free Press*. In 1924 he wrote:

> There are other ways, however, of amusing yourself at the Alpine Club camp than by climbing Mount Robson. One of the most delightful of the expeditions is a three-day trip to Calumet Creek, which I made in company with Dr. F.C. Bell. We started up the main Mount Robson glacier, which flows right down to the camp, but soon left it for a hillside which might have been carried straight over from Scotland and deposited in the middle of the Rockies. The place was pink with the exquisite moss campion. By the side of the streams grew the tall grass of Parnassus; but there was one touch which you never find on a Scottish hill, namely, the great sheets of forget-me-nots of a blue so lovely that it took your breath away.
>
> We passed over the Snowbird Pass where we heard the whistle of the pika, the little policeman of the mountains who blows his whistle so as to inform his friends of the approach of danger, and came out on the great Coleman Glacier. Nothing more pleasant can be imagined than walking on a dry glacier, that is to say, one uncovered by snow. The nails of your climbing boots cut into the rough ice, the going is sufficiently uneven to exercise a great variety of muscles, and there is the constant interest of looking down the crevasses bathed with lovely green light, and the curious round moulins into which the water pours. We crossed the head of the Smoky River Valley down which we had magnificent views, light clouds dappling the hills with floating

shadows, and the snow peaks all around shining into the glorious sunlight. Towards evening we crossed a high ridge, and far below us in the valley we caught sight of the white tents of the little camp by Calumet Creek, whilst a glimpse of the blue smoke from the cook's fire curling up among the trees served to whet our already keen appetites.

The final descent to the camp lay through the most lovely alpland or alpine meadow of which it is possible to conceive. Through the moss carpet flowed little brooks, clear as crystals, and not milky like all glacial torrents. Arising from the green carpet were millions of blue lupins, almost knee high, whilst in lesser abundance but even greater loveliness were red and yellow columbines, blue forget-me-nots (and what a blue!), the scarlet paint brush and the pink patches of the tiny moss campion. It was a Garden of Eden, with not even a mosquito to disturb our happiness.

On the following day we climbed Calumet, a simple snow-and-ice ascent for part of the way, but terminating in a splendid rock arête so narrow that when you sat astride it your left leg hung down a sheer precipice, and your right leg down a slab against which you plastered your fleshly integument whilst your immortal spirit strove ever upwards. Sensational, but perfectly safe and easy. The view from the top was that magnificent tumbled sea of mountain peaks with which we had already become so familiar, and which made us realize, once more, what an unequalled playground are these Canadian Rockies of ours where "heavens are blue above mountains where sleep the unsunned tarns."

About this time he was back in Europe when he climbed the Matterhorn, a picture of which adorned his study wall thereafter. He wrote, "We left for the climb while it was still dark and two hours later the dawn came. . . ."

What of Those of Us Who Are Left?
His views on the War had now mellowed to a realization of the bitterness and the loss. In an Armistice Day address to the students of the Faculty of Medicine on 10 November 1928 he said:

Once again we meet on this day of thinking back and remembering. Ten years have passed, and some of the memories, once so poignant, are beginning to fade. A new generation is growing up who never lived through those terrible years. And yet this day must remain the most solemn in all the year, the most full of meaning for ourselves and for all mankind.

Should it be a day of joy, or of sadness? Who can say? It depends so much on our outlook on life, on our ideas as to what life and death are, and on what is really worthwhile. We know so little.

You remember what Socrates said to the judges who condemned him to death: "The time has come when we must part, and go our respective ways — I to die, and you to live; and which of us has the happier fortune is known to none, except to God."

It is on this day that I think of one of the dearest friends I ever had, brave as a lion, a fellow of infinite charm. He is gone, and his place can never be taken. Some of you here have suffered even deeper loss, which has left a pain that not all the comfort in the world can ever quite still.

We who are gathered here are of many creeds and beliefs. Some find belief easy, others find it hard. Our scientific training and habit of mind do not tend to make it easier. And yet there are some great certainties and verities that we can all lay hands on. And one of these is sacrifice. The scarlet thread of sacrifice runs through life; it ennobles whatever it touches; we see it in the highest form in some of the most sublime manifestations of the human spirit. No matter what our creed, what our faith may be, we recognize that scarlet thread and bow our heads before it. And those boys who have died, what more could they have done for us who remain? "Greater love hath no man than this, that he lay down his life for a friend." And what of us who are left? Have we no duty to those we remember? Surely we have one duty, to swear an oath and keep it that this thing shall not be again — this foul and beastly and cruel and wanton thing that we call war. Easy to say, but how hard to live up to. For when the blasts of war blow in our ears, how can we hearken to the sweet voice of reason? And this is even more true of the nation than of the individual. How easy it is for petty jealousies as well as material interests to come between great nations, how difficult to avoid the irritation engendered by unjust criticism. But why should we mind criticism if we know it to be unjust? There is a great Eastern saying that we may all bear in mind when the little jackals of the press are in full cry: "The dogs may bark, but the caravans move on," and we believe that the caravan of mankind is on the march. Governments make war, but the people can enforce peace.

Are we then never to draw the sword again? I will not say that. We may have to fight to save the weak from oppression, we may have to fight to right the wrong, but for God's sake let us be sure that it is for these high ends that we let loose the dogs of war.

And so on this day of memories we turn our thoughts once more to those who sleep far away in graves that John McCrae has sung of in immortal verse. And after all, it is not a day of sadness but of thankfulness.

> Nothing is here for tears, nothing to wail
> Or knock the breast; nothing but well and fair,
> And what may quiet us in a death so noble.

The mystery remains. Life and death will always remain a mystery. We bow our heads in the two-minutes silence, but we can look up again with bright faces.

> We can smile to think God's greatness flows around our incompleteness,
> Round our restlessness his rest.

The wounds in the soul left by war were healing; the faith that was instilled in Portsoy Free Kirk was fading to agnosticism.

The Black Years

The old Dean died. The new Dean was A.T. Mathers, a psychiatrist. The Depression struck, and with it what seemed a radical deterioration in climate in what was already a cold enough city. The Great Depression of 1929 affected almost every facet of life in Winnipeg. It all started with the 29 October 1929 stock market crash. The prairie drought led to drastic reductions in farm income, and thus in demand for food and services. Unemployment led to large expenditures on relief for the poor. Government appropriations for health and education were reduced. In the fall of 1930 the freight cars were laden with unemployed nomads, criss-crossing the country in a vain search for work. In 1932, twenty percent of the population of Winnipeg was on outdoor relief, sawing tamarack cordwood at the woodyard. There was a clothing famine. The unemployed could not afford food; and prices dropped to the detriment of the purveyors. There was little actual starvation, but much undernutrition and misery. It was to the advantage of those who had a job, or were well off like Boyd, that the price of labour and various materials fell. There is no comment in any of Boyd's letters of his view on the Depression.

In 1931 dust storms darkened the sky, accompanied by plagues of grasshoppers which ate anything that had survived the arid weather. During the month of February in 1936 the thermometer seldom rose above -40°F. It probably reached -50°F but the recording thermometer stuck. Blockheaters were not yet universal, and many automobiles were laid up for the winter. The streets were empty and frigid. Pedestrians scuttled from one building to another, and the wheels of the streetcars squeaked their protests in the cold, as Gray describes.

Temperatures soared to new records in the summer of 1936, reaching 108°F on 11 July 1936, followed by a terrifying thunderstorm. In the same year there were epidemics of polio and sleeping sickness. By early 1937 Winnipeg must have seemed a good place to leave.

For the University of Manitoba, the hardships of the Depression were rendered worse by the sad Machray affair. John Machray KC, revered churchman and lawyer, had become Honorary Bursar of the University of Manitoba in 1903 and financial agent in 1907. He occupied a similar position of trust in the affairs of the Anglican Church as Chancellor of the Archdiocese of Rupertsland. Over the period of his stewardship he embezzled $900,000 from the University and $800,000 from the Church — in each case a large proportion of the fluid assets of the institution. Much of the stolen money came from the Rockefeller Foundation grant.

The inevitable budget reductions came — on 13 June 1933 a ten percent reduction in part-time salaries and a thirty percent reduction in departmental appropriations. In a report to the medical faculty, Dean

Mathers spoke of a forty-three percent failure rate and of a faculty "discouraged almost to the point of rebellion" by the necessity of trying to teach too many students with inadequate space and equipment. A limit on the intake of students followed the Dean's warning.

Silver Linings
Despite the Depression all was not dark. The medical school continued to be well rated as a teaching institution. On 28 August 1933 it was graded A, one of only three in Canada, and its students continued to do well in external qualifying examinations. Meanwhile Boyd's successes were little affected by the dirty economic climate.

The Manitoba Medical College celebrated its jubilee on 14-16 May 1934 amid much academic junketing. Boyd played a leading part. He put on one of his by then very popular clinico-pathologic conferences, and delivered the Memorial Lecture to his predecessor, Gordon Bell. Boyd was now a twenty-year Winnipeg institution built into the bricks. After his trip to Stanford in 1934 he received a salary increase of $360 per year to bring him to the same level as that offered him in California.

Limitation on the admission of Jewish students was now in force. On 7 April 1935, faculty executive minutes record "five students of the Jewish race be admitted to the first year next session. Carried." There is no record that Boyd stood either for or against this racist decision, but while he cannot escape a charge of complicity, he should not carry more blame than other educated people of the time. It was the prejudice of much of the country in which he grew up, as well as the country and time in which he lived his adult life.

Much information on Boyd's life in Winnipeg from 1934 comes from a correspondence he carried on for many years with Dr. F.W. Wiglesworth. He had graduated in Manitoba in 1931 and spent the next two years working with Boyd; he was subsequently appointed pathologist to the Children's Memorial Hospital in Montreal. The letters which Boyd wrote to him over many years give some flavour of his latter days in Winnipeg.

At this stage of his life, Boyd was still an enthusiastic practising pathologist with an interest in the recognition of new lesions, and in the application of new staining methods. He discusses the problems of sharpening microtome knives — ". . . three-in-one oil on the strop and then rub in the rouge." He wrote in November 1933, "We have solved the problem of the surgical sections. You may remember that they used to vary terribly. Now they are always good." In 1934, he was looking for, and found examples of the recently described glomus tumour.

He asked a colleague for material from a Wilms tumour, and from a parotid tumour, and recorded his attempts to stain the pituitary in the new manner — "mucicarmine working beautifully." In 1936 he described "looking over some of the slides which you sent me of thymoma and Schwannoma. . . ." These are words of an eager surgical pathologist. His colleagues at the Winnipeg General Hospital regarded him as such. He still did some autopsies, especially on the bodies of prominent people, like that of a local archbishop.

A junior medical colleague who assisted him at an autopsy in the early 1930s remembers him as "capable, confident and efficient, a lean muscular man with strong hands and firm grip. Except when actually working, he smoked continuously. He was an immensely creative man but considerably dependent on others, for the interpretation of microslides, for example." In 1931 Boyd wrote, "the smooth working of the laboratory is largely due to the willing co-operation of my technicians — Mr. E. Teal and Miss Edna Cockburn, and still more to the efficiency and skill of Dr. Sara Meltzer."

It was a static period, forced upon the medical school by the hard economic times. There were no alterations to the professional staff of either the Hospital or University Departments between 1932 and 1937.

Boyd was enthusiastic in developing the pathological museum which was by this time a focus of student attention. In a spurt of effort in 1933 he requested, and received, more space and help. But he did much of the preparing of the text and photographs for the museum displays himself. He noted, in 1933, "that there was great activity in the Museum. That there will be much more to see next time — gross and microscopic pictures, pictures of clinical states (Addison, Graves, myxoedema etc.), or history of medicine pictures." Many of his gross specimens are still used in teaching medical students in Winnipeg.

He was busy, with not "much time for badminton". His spare time was spent in small convivial gatherings; the pleasures of the whisky bottle became more attractive to the Scot from the manse; it is a familiar consolation in the withering desolation of the prairie cold. A kenspeckle pathologist in another prairie city has characterized prairie life as "tolerable only with an alcohol level of 40".

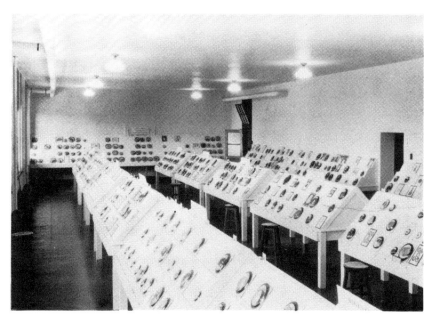

Pathology Museum — Winnipeg

Entertainment was not lacking in Winnipeg — Nijinsky visited with the Russian ballet in 1934. On 22 February 1933 it was recorded that "Horowitz is coming soon and the London String Quartet were here recently." In 1934 visitors included Kreisler playing Rachmaninoff, and the San Carlo Opera Company. Boyd was enthusiastic about acquiring the "most glorious Beethoven records". He sat on the board of the Winnipeg Ballet.

He now travelled a great deal. He visited Washington where he talked to pathologists, the International Association of Medical Museums and the American Society of Physicians. On his return from a trip to Spokane, Washington, he was arranging to visit Vancouver six months later. New York and Atlantic City were other places on his list at this time. In 1934 he was President of the American Association of Pathologists, a powerful professional body. With sure social touch he ordered Drambuie to be served after the President's Dinner; "Drambuie Bill" they called him. In the same year he was President of the International Medical Museums Association. Comfortably and with aplomb he performed the social duties incumbent upon him in his exalted position in the academic world. Even further advancement naturally followed.

The books were beginning to press upon him. He wrote (21 October 1932), "Now that the 3rd ed. of the Surgical Pathology is done I have a feeling of unlimited leisure." The success of the books was giving him great pleasure. He noted, "The textbook is being used in 18 American schools; not bad at the end of 6 weeks." In answer to a query, he wrote in 1934, "Ignore the antediluvian surgical path. . . . look up 'The Textbook'."

His attitudes to teaching were changing. While he still lectured quite extensively, he noted that he had "now reached the stage in our teaching where we have not only dispensed with the lecture, but almost with the microscope. I find that we can use the oil immersion lens for blood films with our new projector, the wonderful new toy."

At different times of the year Boyd lectured to second-year students on general pathology, and third-year students on organ pathology, in each case at two o'clock in the afternoon, a time when students tend to drowse. They did not sleep in Boyd's classes — "He was quite articulate and highly descriptive. He made his subject glow with interest and our attention was held as though we were hypnotized. There was a metal pole from floor to ceiling in the old-fashioned lecture theatre, and when excited Boyd would grasp it hand over hand and climb it. He still had a pronounced Scottish accent, but could not clearly trill an R, and would always talk of 'bwonchiectasis'. When he was asked a question he would drop his eyes to the floor, and then roll his eyes, and one eyebrow would come down."

There was a change in teaching methods, as the years passed, away from the didactic lecture. From about 1927, and certainly by 1933, at the beginning of third year the class was divided into groups of three students. Each group was told what subject matter they should present in turn throughout the year. One student of each group outlined the subject, another summarized recent literature on the subject, while the third student illustrated the material with the microprojector, lantern slides, the epidiascope and specimens from the museum, while the Professor acted as moderator. The presentation was made in a traditional high-rise amphitheatre. Each group was also responsible for attending and assisting at a number of autopsies throughout the year, and presenting the findings to the class.

Boyd enjoyed eating lunch with the interns in the Hospital and reserved the chair at the head of the table. If he couldn't attend, he preferred that the chair not be used. He would pass round his royalty cheques for twenty interns to admire. At first they were interested, then bored. He was a paradoxical mixture of humility and showmanship, always conscious of his status. He remained popular with students, but these quirks of behaviour did not go down well with the more mature junior staff. He mixed well with students and even then took a fair dram. One student remembers him at a party in the Fort Garry Hotel wrestling with his friend "Buzz" Bell, the physician, and tearing up telephone books in the hotel lobby.

His literary output during the Winnipeg years was remarkable. He wrote five textbooks in thirteen years. The books increasingly dominated his life. "The furnace exploded blowing soot through the entire ms of Dr. Boyd's new book." "Smoke was billowing out of the Boyds' house, and Bill ran out into the streets clutching his precious manuscripts." They were lively and industrious years that were not to come again.

Please Don't Go.
Like many another academic settler on the prairie Boyd was always on the lookout for opportunities elsewhere. He was not a member of the

A PETITION

to

DOCTOR WILLIAM BOYD

THAT HE WILL NOT RESIGN AS

Professor of Pathology

of the

University of Manitoba

We, your past students, have learned with mixed feelings that you have been offered the post of Pathologist to Guy's Hospital. It has given us a thrill of pleasure to think of the honor you have won, and in the imagination to contemplate you upholding the great tradition of Guy's Clinician - pathologists. But the thrill gives place to a chill. We wish you not to go. You have brought fame to yourself and to our school. Opportunities for greater fame are to hand; facilities are excellent; life not unpleasant. You have been a stimulus to us, and we fear for serious collapse of the patient should that stimulus be withdrawn.

We, who sign this do so not only in our own names, but in the names of many who cannot be reached in the time available.

[signatures]

Winnipeg, Man., March 2, 1933.

We, the students of the Faculty of Medicine, the University of Manitoba, respectfully wish to tender to William Boyd, M.D., M.R.C.P. (Edin.), F.R.C.P. (Lond.), Dipl. Psych., F.R.S.(C), their warm congratulations on his receipt of a very high honor from Guy's Hospital and London University. Appreciating though we do this high distinction and the opportunity it would offer Dr. Boyd for enlarged usefulness and service in the profession, we are mindful that his acceptance of the honor would inflict an irreparable loss to this University as well as to the wider life of Canada.

We, therefore, respectfully but most earnestly urge Dr. Boyd to consider our deep hope that he may find it possible to remain with the University of Manitoba and to here continue those labors which have won the esteem of students and the profession alike, and which it may be have their best fruition in our new land.

[signatures]

Two petitions — Please don't go!

massive and exclusive British pathological establishment, but by 1930 was well known and respected in the United States. His success was so obvious that offers of jobs in Britain and elsewhere flowed in.

He visited Stanford in 1933 to discuss an appointment, and had an exciting trip down which included his meeting Greta Garbo. "I am still intoxicated with my California experience. The country is wonderful beyond belief and the girls even more so! Flying is the only way to travel. To awaken in the middle of the night and look out on Orion level with the window. . . ." He was enthusiastic about the pleasures of aeroplane flight — and about the "pretty American girls".

On 7 March 1933 a telegram from Guy's Hospital Medical School in London arrived: SOME MEMBERS STAFF GUYS HOSPITAL ANXIOUS LEARN WHETHER YOU WOULD BE LIKELY ACCEPT VACANCY UNIVERSITY CHAIR GUYS IF OFFERED STOP SALARY £1400 PLUS SUPERANNUATION CONYBEARE GUYS HOSPITAL. He also had discussions with McGill University, and notes that he "came within an ace of moving there."

Professor M.J. Stewart wrote on 9 March 1934, to ask "whether you would wish to be considered for the Chair of Pathology at the Postgraduate Medical School in London. Sir Robert Muir is your fervent admirer, and even if one of his own pupils were a candidate, I think he would probably be quite willing to act as a referee for you. Professor L.S.P. Davidson wrote on 9 September 1936 of the Chair of Pathology at the University of Aberdeen "should you apply you would be appointed."

There is no question that several universities negotiated with Boyd and told him that he would be a favoured candidate. It is not so certain from his files how often he was actually offered a post in writing. For his own advantage, Boyd made full political use of these approaches, but could probably have moved before he did, had he wished. His decision to remain in Winnipeg for the time being helped to create the legend which he was already consciously or subconsciously weaving. He resisted for a long time, reacting to the support of his own students who petitioned him to stay. The invitations elsewhere must have made him realize ultimately that Winnipeg was quite small beer. In 1937 he finally accepted an invitation from Toronto. As Dean Gallie showed him around Toronto, he remembered the recent extreme Winnipeg weather.

There were many expressions of regret from students and staff, but this time he was allowed to go. "The Dean suggested that as Dr. Boyd had spent a great deal of time and energy in building up our museum, he thought it would be a courteous act on our part to call the pathological museum in the future, the Boyd Museum. "This was heartily approved" by the executive on 24 September 1937.

When he came to Manitoba he was unknown and possessed of a rather scant knowledge of pathology. He left for Toronto having written several medical best-sellers. His writing exalted the reputation of a little-known medical school. At the same time there was a serious lack of medical research in Winnipeg and Boyd shared the blame. Textbooks and innovative research are not synonymous.

One man at least was devastated when Boyd announced that he was leaving for Toronto:

> I can tell you an example of a 17-year-old high school student, disappointed because of the Depression in his hopes of studying medicine, who dropped casually into the Pathology Department of the Winnipeg General Hospital in search of a job, one day in 1934. Dr. Boyd whom he had never heard of before spent the next hour and a half with him, explaining the various career lines that might be open to a technician and promised to get in touch if any opening occurred. Some three weeks later Dr. Boyd called his home personally one evening to offer a "position" as lab boy in the Dept. of Pathology of the University at $25.00 a month.
>
> In the next three years, the young man happily cleaned, mounted, catalogued museum specimens — the beginnings of the first Boyd "watch-glass museum", collected and returned journals to libraries, engaged under Boyd's stimulus in devising a technique then unknown for staining the Golgi apparatus, projecting the slides at Boyd's undergraduate lectures — and incidentally sitting enthralled at his annual Christmas reading to the Third Year Class, in lieu of a lecture, — Sir Frederick Treves' "Elephant Man", or Kipling's "The Miracle of Purun Bhagat".
>
> Then one day in 1937 the bottom fell out of his world — as near to medicine as he ever hoped to come, when Boyd informed him that he was leaving Manitoba to take the Chair of Pathology in Toronto. The despair was short-lived however, for Boyd added almost immediately, with that characteristic lift of an eyebrow,

"and when I leave I would like to put up the money in order for you to study medicine."

This he did — and over the next five years, by correspondence or on the occasion of his visits to Winnipeg, kept a close eye on progress, kindly chiding and encouraging when required, usually at his protégé's inabilities in English which understandably Boyd felt to be more important than Anatomy or Chemistry. On graduation this spiritual son of William Boyd went on to follow his mentor's first medical interest — psychiatry.

The writer knows well of Boyd's intense feelings and concerns for colleagues and staff, and to his deep commitment to the human values of gallantry, loyalty and courage. But because he rarely spoke of his material gifts, one has no idea how many young people he helped in the way described above.

For this one instance I can vouch for the verity. For I was that young man.

The author of this letter, who attained high academic success in medicine, will remain anonymous.

Boyd's characteristic farewell to Manitoba was an elegant little essay in the *University of Manitoba Medical Journal*, entitled "On the Dangers of Scrappiness":

Our fathers and grandfathers were brought up to appreciate the value of thoroughness. We admire it in them and in their writings. The Victorians knew their reading, writing and arithmetic. But it was much easier for them than for us. The conditions of modern life make for diffuseness and scrappiness. There is a modern craze for news. Not only are there newspapers, or rather sheets of advertisements amongst which snippets of information are scattered here and there, but there are weekly news magazines containing so much information that by the time you have finished one issue the next is arriving, whilst the radio in the intervals of crooning gives us news from all parts of the world. Now, news is one of the most interesting of things. The newspaper man calls it a story, and he is right. But it has its dangers. You may remember that when Paul came to Athens he found that the people were always seeking after some new thing. Yes, but that was after the Golden Age had passed away. News is delightful for the old, for the businessman who has nothing to do with his evenings, for the feeble-minded. But for the student it is a seducer whose danger is its apparent innocence. It fills the mind with scraps of information, but the student's aim and ideal should be thoroughness, not scrappiness. It is thoroughness which makes a man a great golfer or figure skater, a great internist or anatomist. But thoroughness and distraction do not go together. I have seen a man studying (?) in a room in which the radio was playing! Such men always feel aggrieved when the list of supplementals comes out.

Another cause of modern scrappiness of mind is the "digest habit". On every bookstall you will see a digest of this and a digest of that, handy little magazines which can be slipped into a pocket or carried on a streetcar. In these places they are splendid, and they will enable you to produce scraps of literary information at a dinner party like a conjurer produces rabbits from a hat. But they have no place in a student's study. His time and the integrity of his mind are too precious. For they do not take the place of the books they abstract. Recently I read a "digest" of *An American Doctor's Odyssey*, and afterwards I read the book itself. The impression created on my mind was absolutely different in the two cases. Imagine reading a digest of *King Lear* or *The Forsyte Saga* or *The Seven Pillars of Wisdom*! Besides, if you are always taking things predigested, what is going to happen to your own digestive organs? May I suggest to the students of our medical school that great pleasure and satisfaction is to be derived from knowing one thing really well, from being master of one subject however small. Thoroughness rather than scrappiness. And with that thoroughness will come competence and mastery, and such mastery will bring the recognition from his fellows which every man enjoys. As Emerson says: "Let a man preach a better sermon, write a better book, or build a better mousetrap than his neighbour — though he build his house in the woods, the world will make a path to his door."

A thorough knowledge of a subject is possible in two branches of thought, the one professional, the other general. The medical student may set himself to become an expert on the anatomy, histology, and physiology of an organ, or on the pathology and clinical features of a disease. The former is more likely to appeal to him in his earlier years, the latter in the clinical part of his course. Should a man interest himself in such an organ as the kidney, prostate or parathyroid, he will be surprised how frequently new information regarding his pet subject meets his eye. The "news" may be scrappy, but it will be integrated in the mind so as to form part of a composite whole. The same is true of a disease such as coronary occlusion, cholecystitis, or bronchogenic carcinoma.

In the field of general reading a student may also become an expert. It is remarkable how, in a very few years, one can read all the works of an author that are worth reading, and when the author is a master of matter or style, these insensibly colour the mind of the reader. But such reading can only be done if one is aware of the danger of scrappiness. *Paradise Lost* and *The Ring and the Book* may appear alarming because of their length, but in my third year in medicine at Edinburgh I read the twelve books of Milton's immortal work on Sunday afternoons before Christmas and the twelve books of Browning after Christmas.

Each man has to decide for himself what he wants, but there is not time in the study of medicine to colour the mind with Robert Louis Stevenson or Conrad, as well as the latest gossip from Hollywood. "Do you know," says Ruskin, "if you read this, that you cannot read that — that what you lose today you cannot gain tomorrow? Will you go and gossip with your housemaid or your stableboy, when you may talk with queens and kings, or flatter yourself that it is with any worthy consciousness of your own claims to respect that you jostle with the hungry and common crowd for entrée here and audience there, when all the while this eternal court is open to you, with its society wide as the world, multitudinous as its days, the chosen and the mighty of every place and time?"

Great books are the greatest relaxation that the world can offer to the hard worked medical man, be he student or practitioner. In his brief moments of leisure he can turn to the great silent company who stand on his bookshelves waiting to be heard. "For a man's true life for which he consents to live may lie altogether in the field of infancy. The clergyman, in his spare hours, may be winning battles, the farmer sailing ships, the banker reaping triumph in the arts; all leading another life, plying another trade from that they chose. For to look at the man is but to court deception. We shall see the trunk from which he draws his nourishment; but he himself is above and abroad in the green dome of foliage, hummed through by winds and nested in by nightingales. For no man lives in the external truth, among salts and acids but in the warm phantasmagoric chamber of his brain, with the painted windows and the storied walls."

If you know your Robert Louis Stevenson you will know where that comes from, as well as dozens of other passages which will become part and parcel of your mind. But such knowledge will never come if you abandon yourself to scrappiness.

It was a repeated theme; at a graduates' farewell dinner on 19 March 1931 at the Fort Garry Hotel he had emphasized, "If you are going to succeed in medicine, you must not let your mind stray," and pointed up the message with a verse likely to appeal to a young, largely male audience:

They gathered up Adolphus with a shovel and a rake
For he had grasped a silken knee, when he should have grasped the brake.

― Chapter 8 ―

Papers, Books and Words

BY 1937 BOYD had reached the peak of his career. His main books were written and what was to come was largely revision and repetition. If William Boyd had never written a book, he would have been a competent professor and hospital pathologist, noted for his vivid turn of phrase as a teacher and after-dinner speaker, and would have accompanied his peers into oblivion. But he is remembered at least for a little longer because he wrote many books that were successful in the marketplace; two of them, fifty years after their first publication, are still being updated by other hands.

Boyd started to contribute to the medical literature at an early stage in his career. His first papers, from 1910 to 1920, relate in the main to neurology, psychiatry and the cerebrospinal fluid. They were competent, but not remarkable.

With a Field Ambulance at Ypres
The First World War gave him something stark and terrible to describe, and he rose to the occasion. His family, like the families of many other young men, must have pressed him to publish the letters he wrote from Ypres. His first book, *With a Field Ambulance at Ypres*, was the result. It was written and published not long after he reached Winnipeg; it was

well reviewed, both locally and across the continent, and led to many invitations to speak on his war experiences. He achieved significant status in a war-engrossed country, and later in a profession where war experience was a necessary ticket of admission to the new medical establishment.

The reviewers made it clear that the young professor had an unusual talent that must be nurtured. Boyd carefully preserved the reviews in a little leather-bound album and must have seen, at least as through a glass darkly, the path he was to tread.

The Cerebrospinal Fluid

Boyd's early work on the cerebrospinal fluid broke no new ground, but led to a systematic review of the subject in his first medical book, *Physiology and Pathology of the Cerebrospinal Fluid* (New York: Macmillan, 1920). It was to some extent the product of a man who had not yet decided whether he wanted to spend his life as a pathologist.

It is an expansion of his MD thesis and gives a succinct account of the cerebrospinal fluid, its examination and its alteration in disordered states. The book was dedicated "To my teacher and chief Byron Bramwell". The author had spent a considerable period, first in asylum practice and later in Winnipeg, investigating the CSF, and could refer to several of his own published articles, so that it was a reasonably authoritative text, simply written, but without the colourful writing that was to follow.

There is a surprising amount of information in the book on clinical neurology. Lumbar puncture was used therapeutically in uraemic coma and eclampsia, and to relieve headache in anaemia, deafness, tinnitus and auditory vertigo, and even convulsions in children. Meningococcal meningitis was treated by instilling antiserum into the cerebrospinal fluid, while tuberculin was instilled in tuberculous meningitis. Neurosyphilis was treated by intravenous injections of Salvarsan, and subsequent injection of the patient's serum containing Salvarsan into the subarachnoid space. The book was recommended by the Professor to the Winnipeg medical students — a captive audience.

During the period ending in 1924, Boyd wrote several long pathologic articles, establishing at once an information base of practical knowledge of morbid anatomy, and a stock of knowledge for his next book. By 1922 he had probably become clear in his mind that his career was

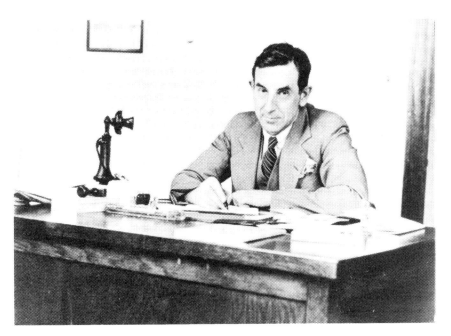
Writing the books

to be as a medical writer. But this needed a foundation of personal experience and original observation before it could be credible.

His long paper on the gall bladder was of some transient significance, but his major original work lies in his authoritative and detailed papers on the Winnipeg encephalitis epidemics. These were important contributions to the literature, widely quoted at the time.

By 1925, when he was forty years old he had made his original contribution to knowledge, the rest was textbooks. He was to say in old age, with uncharacteristic modesty, that he had made no significant original contribution to science; but he had put new bricks on the pyramid of science, smaller than those of many scientists, but larger than those of most.

Surgical Pathology

In 1925, his first major medical book appeared — *Surgical Pathology*, published by W.B. Saunders with 349 illustrations and 13 coloured plates. He had by now won some acceptance in scientific circles of the country of his adoption; the title page reveals that he was now a Fellow of the Royal Society of Canada.

The book was specifically directed at surgeons and written in a discursive tone, although it was immediately prescribed reading for Manitoba medical students. At the beginning of Chapter 1, Boyd described the need for a surgeon to have a good knowledge of pathology. The prose was now ringing.

> The surgery of today is based on pathology. Unless he builds on that solid foundation the surgeon is no better than a hewer of flesh and a drawer of blood.
>
> It has not always been so. We do not need to look far into the dark backward and abysm of time to realize that the foundation of surgery was the sand of empiricism rather than the bed rock of pathology.

He describes in some detail the attempts made to produce anti-cancer vaccines from bacterial cultures, the then well-known "Coley's Fluid". As was common at that time, he believed that they were of some value.

Inflammation, syphilis, tuberculosis, gangrene (dry and wet) — all the old diseases are there described in a clear, though superficial way.

There is little obscure theorizing about causation. The descriptions are gripping. On healing: "should anything interfere with the onward march of the epithelium. . . ." The lesion of erysipelas "[has a margin like] the burnt edge of a smouldering sheet of paper." Anthrax: "I saw a most characteristic example of malignant pustule in France on the face of a soldier who had used his sheepskin coat as a pillow, and who had a slight abrasion on the cheek."

When he did not know, he said so. On the cause of tumours: ". . . the essential cause is still unknown; the veil covering the mystery has not yet been rent in twain. . . . Theory after theory cometh up as a flower, only in turn to be cut down like the grass." There is the ring of the Portsoy pulpit.

In the rest of the book, he describes the pathology of organs of special concern to the surgeon. In those days, patients went to the doctor when disease was well established. An illustration of "early" carcinoma of lip was a lesion we would now regard as advanced. In the gall bladder "the graceful, fragile gossamer folds of mucosa are completely altered in appearance, being loaded down by dense yellow opaque masses, much as a delicate birch tree might be weighed down by a load of snow." He describes carcinoma of the appendix as a common tumour, referring to 225 reported autopsy cases, but notes its benign behaviour. The lesion would now be labelled carcinoid. The account of carcinoma of the colon, now a common disease, is inadequate even for its day. But he was writing on the basis of seven years' experience — that of a newly qualified staff pathologist by today's standards. He quoted beliefs of the day that have since been discredited: that hypernephromas (carcinomas of the kidney) arose in adrenal tissue; that cancer cells permeate lymphatics rather than spread along them by embolism; and that many deaths under anaesthesia were due to status thymolymphaticus, no longer accepted as a pathologic entity.

The microscopic descriptions are in places very sketchy, and there are some subjects about which the professor did not yet know very much, glioma for instance. The old surgical eponyms are still there — Pott's disease of the spine and Pott's puffy tumour — to remind us that the pathology that he saw in his practice in Winnipeg in the early 1920s was still little changed from that seen by Percival Pott in the 18th Century. Myeloma was "a curious and rare condition" and "gonorrhoeal arthritis is a common disease." In 1992, gonococcal arthritis is uncommon because of improved treatment, not improved morals, and myeloma is common because enough people survive to contract it.

While still unknown in the wide world of pathology, he had spent a weekend on the Mayos' houseboat, and at the suggestion of his young assistant, Daniel Nicholson, he asked Will Mayo to write a foreword to *Surgical Pathology*. "What is needed today," Mayo wrote, "in the literature of surgical pathology is a work that will serve as a handbook to the surgeon, and the internist, and a guide to the beginner in the field of medicine. Dr. Boyd has made an earnest effort to fill this need. His book is didactic in tone, as is necessary in a volume of this scope, not judicial, fortunately, because to be judicial one must deal only with proved facts and give no play to scientific imagination. It is a sincere attempt to place pathology before the student and the practitioner from the practical standpoint." So wrote William J. Mayo. It was not highly enthusiastic, but it served to support Boyd's first attempt at writing a pathology book.

The Pathology of Internal Disease

He must have started on the next book, *The Pathology of Internal Disease*, soon after packing *Surgical Pathology* off to the publisher. In its sixth and seventh editions it was called, more appropriately, *Pathology for the Physician*. This book was published not by Saunders, but by Lea & Febiger in 1931.

It is a comprehensive and discursive account of those diseases which are found in the medical wards of a teaching hospital, or which would be included in a course of study for one of the higher examinations in Internal Medicine. It is illustrated with 298 engravings, pictures of gross specimens, and photomicrographs, most of rather high quality for the period.

Boyd sets out in his preface to define his purpose — to teach medicine, not pathology. "In the preface of Rokitansky's great work on Pathological Anatomy, written in 1846, there occurs this sentence: 'While engaged in working out the design of this Pathological Anatomy I have throughout endeavoured to act the part of a clinical teacher.' The author . . . has allowed himself to wander rather freely in the realms of pathological physiology." Throughout the book there is ample space given to the clinical course of disease, often with long quotations from masterly original descriptions. The microscopic descriptions are used to explain disease, not as ends in themselves.

The text has become dated less than might be expected sixty years later. The emphasis on bacterial disease, tuberculosis and syphilis would now seem inappropriate; but most of the material is still remarkably accurate. The accounts are discursive summaries of what experienced physicians carry around in the backs of their minds, and errors inappropriate to the day are hard to find.

By its prose style this and his other major books stand out from most other modern medical texts. The author rejoices, without apology, in the beauty of the English language and sees no reason why a medical textbook should not benefit from it. The first sentence of the first chapter reads: "Of all the ailments which blow out life's little candle, heart disease is the chief." When a patient dies of heart failure without demonstrable cause: "Such cases may be put down to shock, status thymolymphaticus or visitation from God." "I have seen a patient walk into hospital with a pericardium literally bulging with pus." At the crisis of resolution in lobar pneumonia: "The sickle of death may come very near." He sometimes quotes himself verbatim: "[Influenza] travels at an extraordinary speed, but not quicker, as is sometimes imagined, than the speed of man. It crosses a continent as fast as an express train, the ocean at the rate of an Atlantic liner, and the desert as slowly as a camel caravan." Not surprisingly, the book was a success.

He included few personal recollections of war. It is a little surprising that he was so restrained in giving clinical examples from the trenches to support the descriptions of morbid changes in human tissue. But by now time's passage had mercifully thrown a veil over images of the past.

A consideration of the reasons for the increase in bronchial carcinoma listed possible causes: "All sorts of irritants including cigarettes. . . . All of these seem highly improbable." Doll's classical epidemiological studies on the relationship between smoking and lung cancer were years in the future.

He opens the chapter on renal disease: "It is now just one hundred years since there was admitted into Guy's Hospital under the care of Richard Bright an intemperate sailor by the name of John King suffering from edema, scanty urine and albuminuria." There follows Bright's account of nephritis.

Textbook of Pathology
Remarkably, the next book appeared as soon as one year later, in 1932.

It was what Boyd regarded as his masterpiece, the *Textbook of Pathology*, also published by Lea & Febiger. It was, like *Pathology of Internal Disease*, explicitly directed to one segment of the profession, in this case medical students. It had 287 engravings and a coloured plate.

The man was now becoming confident in his stance. "A speaker, whatever his subject, must keep his audience in mind, otherwise he is lost." Despite his aim to teach medicine he was unapologetic about what was now his own trade — he had been a pathologist for 15 years. "Morbid anatomy is not dead and never has been, except in the hands of those whose dull minds would take the breath of life from the most vital subject."

The book has a clear pattern. It is oriented primarily to the methods of diagnosis of human disease. Symptoms are recounted, followed by a description of the morbid anatomy, ending in an attempt to correlate these according to contemporary understanding of disease processes. There is considerable discussion of disordered physiology and quite frequent admissions of ignorance or even of his having been wrong in past writings. The book is never complicated, partly because of clear exposition, but also because of a tendency to bypass difficult problems. In the traditional pattern, Part I is on general pathology and Part II on special pathology.

He had little time for immunology: "The saying that ignorance, however aptly veiled in an attractive terminology, remains ignorance, is particularly applicable to the science of immunology." Some of his prejudices were more picturesque than sustainable: "Beer and such red wine as port are much more dangerous than whisky; for this reason gout is a rare disease in Scotland." On the whole, however, the text was factually reliable.

Patches of vivid human interest capture the attention. On epidemic encephalitis (lethargica) he wrote:

> Winnipeg was visited by two epidemics, the first in the winter of 1919-20, the second at the beginning of 1923. In the first epidemic the patient was dull, lethargic, somnolent, and showed oculomotor disturbances. He would lie like a log in bed with drooping lids or closed eyes, the lines of expression all ironed out, sunk in a stupor which no external stimuli could penetrate, the flash and speed of the mind gone, the dim rushlight of

reason hardly flickering. In the second epidemic the picture had changed completely. Body and mind were now keyed to full activity. The muscles were in a state of constant movement, which was paralleled by a condition of mental excitement. Occupation formed the main topic of conversation: the teacher was continually teaching, the merchant was casting up accounts, the builder planning new houses. The first picture was akinetic, the second hyperkinetic.

The book is replete with good clinical descriptions and good descriptions of gross anatomy; it is clearly an undergraduate text, and not a graduate textbook intended to help physician or surgeon towards differential diagnosis or the acquisition of higher diplomas.

The *Textbook* sold like hot cakes: the author wrote that "it was being used in 18 American medical schools; not bad at the end of 6 weeks." The first edition was 20,000 copies.

The Introduction to Medical Science
The Introduction to Medical Science was the last of the books conceived and written during Boyd's Winnipeg years. It was published, in 1937, also by Lea & Febiger, who now clearly understood that they were on to a good thing. Boyd was by now a Fellow of the Royal College of Physicians in London. It was the turn of the London medical establishment to accept him.

The book was 300 pages long and, illustrated with 108 engravings, it gave an "aeroplane view of disease." It was written for the nurse, premedical student and hospital technician, and attempted to give a "dynamic and functional rather than static and anatomical" account. "A little knowledge is a dangerous thing, but not if you know how little it is."

The treatment was cursory, yet clear, relating real life to cells and the watery fluid in which they live. "Hunger can be endured for several days; thirst is unendurable." Then follows T.E. Lawrence's description from the *Seven Pillars of Wisdom* of death from thirst in the desert. The language is vivid as ever.

On syphilis: "Tertiary lesions are so widespread that to enumerate them would be like giving the list of the ships in the *Iliad* or the names of the kings of Judah."

In 1937 Boyd left Winnipeg; his literary output had been enormous for a man whose life was mainly devoted to teaching and to the practice of pathology. In twenty-two years, he wrote five books. After leaving Winnipeg he was to write nothing more of major importance. (Please see Appendix 2.)

Shortly after he left for Toronto, a lecturing visit to the University of Kansas School of Medicine led to another little book, *Lectures in Pathology*, published by the Extension Division of that university. It is a neat little reprint of his lectures, as readable as ever. It did not have a wide circulation.

The Spontaneous Regression of Cancer
The Michigan Pathological Society invited him to deliver the Weller Lecture at the University of Michigan, Ann Arbor, in 1965. This led to his last book, *The Spontaneous Regression of Cancer* (Springfield: Thomas, 1966).

It is a sunset book, written by a master of the language, but now a little more verbose than he might have been when younger. At eighty years he could write an elegant contribution summarizing the reports of others on an interesting subject which had not previously been considered in such detail.

The Golden Chain
Boyd spent much time revising and updating his books; in many ways he was their prisoner, fastened to them by a golden chain. They were his children and he loved them, even his least favourite *Surgical Pathology*. As early as 1933 he commented adversely on it in a letter to a friend; in 1955 he noted in the preface to the seventh edition that it had begun to show its age, and he acknowledged that others had helped to correct some of the more glaring errors. A comparison of the 1925 and 1955 editions shows much new material, new pictures, text and references. Of all his family, the *Textbook of Pathology* was his favourite — "The Textbook" as he called it.

He leaned on others, sometimes with generous acknowledgement, sometimes with none. A presentation copy of the 1965 edition of *Pathology for the Physician*, given to Dr. John Barrie, bears the manuscript note, "I hope that the entire next edition will bear your name." He sometimes re-used passages from his own previous writings, but on the whole the books were written separately with appropriate material for distinct audiences. There is in the (1965) *Pathology for the Physician* a good up-to-date account of water and electrolyte metabolism, a difficult subject for a man who was essentially an anatomic pathologist; and there is some vintage Boyd on the same subject. "Water is the fabric of everything that lives. The baby consists mostly of water, whilst the old man or woman shrivels up like a wilted plant." He had learned the use of pictures, and cut material that was no longer topical. Coverage of encephalitis, which had never recurred on the scale of the epidemics in the 1920s, shrank from twelve pages to one and a half.

The 8th edition (1970) of the *Textbook of Pathology* bore the subtitle "Structure and Function in Disease" and had been considerably rewritten in a brave attempt to keep up with the pathology of its day. "Old diseases are passing away . . . but new ones are continually taking their place. . . . The inn that shelters for the night is not the journey's end." The consensus of the reviewers was that, while the book still had the Boyd magic, it was not quite so up-to-date as newer books, nor as books revised by a group of authors. A new edition rewritten by Dr. A.C. Ritchie was published in 1990.

The *Introduction to Medical Science*, published in 1952, has pictures of better quality, more on immunology, and a brief account of the history of medicine. It was to be radically rewritten in 1977 by Dr. H. Sheldon.

Words
Boyd's views on writing and the use of words were crystallized in an after-dinner talk which he gave on many occasions, in different forms. Much of it is derivative, largely from Sir Ernest Gowers' *Plain Words*, and its popularity tells as much perhaps about Boyd's success in choosing audiences as his skill in choosing words. But excerpts tell us something about the man; they are from a version given to the American Association of Pathologists and Bacteriologists in Cleveland in 1951 and entitled "Words".

> There are of course all sorts of words. There are good words and bad words. You may remember the old lady who congratulated Samuel Johnson: "I am glad that you made such a thorough search for them." There are of course in reality no good words or bad words, for there is nothing either good or bad but thinking makes it so.

Whatever else you may do, you will always be using words. For words are the tools of thought, and you will often find that you are thinking badly because you are using the wrong tools. (The power and pleasure of words are enduring, and can be enjoyed by all men. They are not the privilege of wealth or intellect or costly education.)

The words of the speaker or writer are the notes of the musician, and you know that by the appropriate choice, arrangement, spacing and accenting of notes the result may be the worst Tin Pan Alley or the most exquisite Mozart concerto. . . .

Everyone is concerned with words, but to pathologists they are of special importance. We write articles and books. We put our ideas into reports and protocols. And we have to speak at conferences and meetings, and also to listen with pleasure or in pain.

We think that we are concerned with facts. To a degree that is true. But concepts far transcend facts, and a concept without words is like a body without flesh. . . .

If you read the works of the masters you get a feeling for words, their meaning and subtlety, their music and magic, just as happens when you listen repeatedly to the masters of music. And there is magic and music in prose as well as in poetry. This was written in Scotland: "There is no sunlight in the poetry of exile. There is only mist, wind, rain, the cry of hill birds and the slow clouds damp above moorland." This is a description of the Scottish War Memorial: "The Edinburgh Shrine is a lament in stone, the greatest of all Scotland's laments, with all the sweetness of pipes crying among hills, with all the haunting beauty of a lament, all the pride, all the grandeur. . . ."

There followed a long quotation from the parable of the prodigal son, words "as simple as the phrases of Mozart's music. Both are the greatest in the world."

The essay shows at once a supple but firm grasp of the English language, a mind rooted in Christian scripture, and a spirit which had left Scotland but still hearkened to it. The papers, the books and the words point back, before his time at medical school in Edinburgh, to an unusually early literary education, leaving a hunger for more.

Easy. A manuscript with few changes

The Travails of Writing
He wrote at first with difficulty, rewriting frequently; his younger colleagues told of trouble interpreting and editing his earlier manuscripts. However, the manuscript of the first edition of the *Introduction to Medical Science* shows rather few alterations. He told of the travail of authorship in a speech given during a university exchange tour in November 1930, to Saskatoon, Edmonton and Vancouver:

> One of the reasons why I am enjoying this trip is that I have just finished a five-year task. I feel that I am on a real holiday. Some five years ago I spent a month in a bed in an Edmonton hospital, and as I had nothing to do, in a weak moment I conceived the idea of writing a book. At first it was great fun planning the lines along which it would develop, and so on, but it was far greater fun finishing the blamed thing off, and shoving it in the mail. You come home tired in the evening, and find the beastly thing lying on your desk with some knotty problem awaiting solution — you feel ready to weep just like Jonah . . . there was only one person hated the thing more than I did and that was my wife.
>
> Then the proofs began to come in, 830 pages of galley proofs, every word to be read with care, then 830 pages of page proofs, all to be read for fresh mistakes, and then the whole thing to be gone over again in order to make the index. By this time it sounded like drivel. After the proofs comes the review; which is worst it is hard to say.

The reviews usually praised highly, and Boyd would celebrate the appearance of a book with a champagne party in his office.

Many Canadian academic pathologists were critical and prescribed different reading for their students. In 1939, when performing his duties as a Visiting Professor at Queen's University, Kingston, he was introduced as having had a meteoric career like a great bird, soaring through space, dropping text books behind him. There was an implication as to the nature and value of the droppings. In Britain, his books for post-graduates were more successful than those for undergraduates, where the market was mainly held by the British pathological establishment, who could impose their texts on their flocks of obedient students. In 1949, Professor A.C.

Lendrum of Dundee, a pillar of British academic pathology, said to his students: "To learn after-dinner speaking, read Boyd; to learn pathology, read Sir Robert's [Muir's] book." In several medical schools, whichever author was prescribed, the students read Boyd.

Like all successful authors he was plagiarized. A hospital in the southern United States kept nagging its staff to publish. The radiologist, tiring of petty tyranny, told his secretary to type out the chapter on bone pathology in Boyd's textbook and submit it to some journal or other. It was accepted and his friends said they understood he had written a good paper. A year or two later the chief of staff approached the radiologist again, asking for more. The radiologist agreed, told his typist to copy the same chapter, and send it to the same journal. It was published and his friends said, "I hear your second paper is even better than your first." A short time afterwards Boyd was revising the section on bone. In the middle of studying an article he lifted his head and said to Enid, "This fellow writes well." But then he came to the phrase, "The bones look as if they had been twisted by a giant hand," and the source of the article came home to him. Characteristically, he wrote to the editor thanking him for the double compliment. By this time the radiologist had died, probably from laughter.

John Barrie, his friend of over thirty years has tried to analyze his success. "The books sold because they were eminently readable. Their style was simple and vivid. Their breadth and humanity dispelled the smell of the morgue. In many editions, they sold worldwide in large numbers and brought him fame and fortune. [In Sheffield] whenever I lectured, they rather resented my efforts to gain their attention and frequently a hand would go up: 'But please sir, Boyd says. . . .' It doesn't matter what textbook you recommend, they will all read Boyd. . . . Look at some of the sources of Boyd's literary style, his great output, and his popularity. For much of his style we are indebted to his mother, for it was she who introduced him to good literature — what the British critic John Ruskin called 'the company of the dead'."

Were Boyd's books good books? They were readable, reasonably accurate and, at least up to about 1965, well researched for their day. Any errors were usually corrected in later editions. None was specifically written as a text for pathologists; they were intended to teach medical students and post-graduate clinicians pathology, and this they did well. Many, many medical students bought them, read them, liked them, and learned the basics of medicine from them. Boyd's files contain many letters from grateful students, often from the Indian sub-continent, and frequently written in tones of adulation; he answered them all. The books contained little that was controversially new or original, except perhaps for the account of encephalitis; elementary texts are places for the accepted canon of knowledge. They represented what an experienced, conventional teacher of pathology believed physicians should know. They were good books, widely read.

Harvard medical students paid Boyd the ultimate accolade. When he visited Harvard, the medical librarian said to him, "We can't keep your books on the shelf. The students steal them." Toronto medical students were put on a diet of Boyd's "Textbook", soon after he went to Toronto. The Toronto medical class was large, which doubtless helped sales, but medical schools all over North America and in many other parts of the world recommended the *Textbook of Pathology* to their students. Boyd's life in Toronto and later was dominated by the need to keep the books up to date.

Chapter 9

The Zenith and the Shadow

THE ZENITH of Boyd's career was his period as Professor and Head of Pathology in the University of Toronto. Here he first felt the chill shadow of his personal evening. Moving from Winnipeg to Toronto in 1937 was a big step up. The city was large and more sophisticated. The population stood at about three quarters of a million, but it was still possible to live near the centre at reasonable cost. From 1930 to 1945 a housing slump held the population constant, but after the Second World War it increased rapidly, due to immigration. In 1950, about the time Boyd retired, the population was 1,100,000, rising to 1,800,000 by the middle 1960s.

Toronto had been Toronto the Good, high Victorian in its contrasts, Casa Loma to Cabbagetown. Despite the Depression it was a rich city. At the beginning of the 1930s the Royal York and the Bank of Commerce were, respectively, the largest hotel and the tallest building in the British Empire. Department stores like Eaton's and Simpson's were palaces of riches. Women were emancipated; knee-length skirts replaced flowing dresses and yards of petticoat. Middle-class households had electric irons, vacuum cleaners and refrigerators, and the ice wagon was slowly disappearing from the streets. By the 1930s more than a million motor cars were on Canadian streets, and it was possible to drive to Hamilton on a reasonably good road, but bearded rag-and-bone men still trundled their carts round the streets collecting household discards.

It was not an uncultured city. The Group of Seven was painting and the Canadian Authors Association was promoting Canadian nationalism in the arts and letters. Three quarters of a million people supported by far the best symphony orchestra in Canada. The Royal Ontario Museum was the biggest and best in the country. There was a very good art gallery; four daily papers were published in what was the centre of the Canadian publishing industry.

Even in the 1930s it was still Toronto the Good. "Constables with stopwatches in the wings of the Royal Alexandra Theatre, timing the kisses . . . ready to ring down the curtain if they lasted more than 20 seconds . . . a mournful Scottish version of America . . . this sanctimonious icebox," lamented Wyndham Lewis.

The drought across the country during the years 1930-1936 affected the prosperity of Toronto, although not as badly as it hurt the West. With drought came depression, unemployment and social confrontation. The average annual salary was $927 while the lowest was $52 for a domestic servant. Soap cost 5 cents a bar, hamburger 5 cents a pound, and the best sirloin 25 cents a pound. A return rail trip to Vancouver required an outlay of $54.25; many destitute men chose to ride the box-cars; poliomyelitis recurred annually. People in Toronto as elsewhere in the 1930s tried to ignore the outside world, which went without intermission from depression to rumours of war. War clouds lowered — the invasion of China, of Abyssinia, the Spanish Civil War.

Doctors were important people. One hundred miles from Toronto medicine was practised in a different and distant world. Country GPs harnessed their teams for a two-hour drive in the middle of a winter night. Their patients still died of pneumonia and tuberculosis in large numbers; and pernicious anaemia had been conquered only recently.

The University of Toronto Medical School
The University of Toronto was a large and important institution. God was on top, personified by Archdeacon Henry John Cody (Anglican), rector of St. Paul's, serving first as Chancellor, then as President. Lester Pearson was teaching history. The University of Toronto Medical School was a relatively large and wealthy school, still basking in the afterglow of the insulin discovery in 1921. There were many distinguished profes-

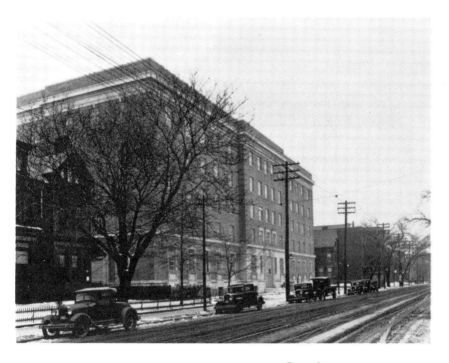

Banting Institute — Toronto, Ontario

sors. J.C.B. Grant and A.W. Ham in Anatomy were writing their respective best-selling texts. G.F. Marrian was to become Professor of Biochemistry. C.H. Best was Professor of Physiology, and Sir Frederick Banting vigorously pursued his research, if with less dramatic effect than in 1921, in the Institute which carried his name. In the 1940s the school was involved in the manufacture of penicillin, and reports of major advances in cardiac surgery had begun to appear.

E.W. Gallie, the dynamic Professor of Surgery, was determined to find the best man to fill the Chair of Pathology, left vacant by the untimely death of Oskar Klotz. Gallie thought very highly of Boyd, and succeeded in persuading him where others had failed. Enid wrote during their visit to Toronto in December 1936 that "he has gone out this morning with Dr. Gallie who is trying to make him see that Toronto is the place to live."

It is not quite certain why the University of Toronto succeeded in attracting Boyd. It was not a matter of salary. The sum offered by Toronto was not much more than his Winnipeg salary; besides, his books had by now made him independently wealthy. In 1947, he was paid $7000 a year at a time when the Professor of Surgery was earning about $20,000. Boyd's royalties brought his income to a similar level.

The offer of sophisticated equipment was not in those days such a draw as it would be now. All Boyd insisted on was a micro-projector and a high-reflectance screen. Perhaps he moved because he was feeling stifled in Winnipeg; he wrote on 26 January 1937, "It was an awful wrench. Things have become too easy for me here, leading to fatty degeneration of the soul." While Toronto had more glamour and status than Winnipeg, it was not quite up to the level of Guy's or Stanford, at both of which, according to Boyd, he had turned down offers of chairs of pathology. Probably his wife did not want to leave Canada; his friend and classmate, J.C.B. Grant the anatomist, was in Toronto and Grant's wife Catriona was Enid's sister. The extraordinarily bad weather in Depression Winnipeg might well have contributed to his decision to move.

The First Ten Years

A little light on Boyd's first days in Toronto is cast by the records of the Department of Pathology. Departmental meetings were held in the evenings and consisted of short papers followed by discussion. Klotz chaired his last meeting on 20 April 1936 and on 18 January 1937 appears the entry: "The morning papers would carry the announcement that

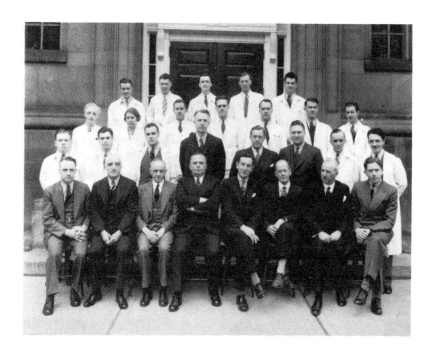

Banting Institute 1938-39 (Courtesy of Toronto Academy of Medicine)
Department of Pathology and Bacteriology:

Front row	2nd row	3rd row	4th row
I.H. Erb	A.J. Blanchard	M.S. Thompson	M.G. Whillans
George Shanks	D.R.E. MacLeod	Mary I. Tom	H. Hayward
Eric A. Linell	D.E.O. Magner	G.D.M. Boddington	J.G. Mickler
W.L. Robinson	E.J. Clifford	R.E. Will	(student
Wm. Boyd	P.H. Greey	J.H. Rickard	demonstrator)
W.L. Holman	W.M. Wilson	M.R. Shaver	F.P. Dewar
Wm. Magner	L.M. Gray	D.B. MacLaren	C.L. Burke
G. Lyman Duff	A.W. Bagnall		

Missing: — Dr. R. Margarite Price

Prof. Wm. Boyd had accepted the invitation of the University of Toronto to occupy the Chair of Pathology."

Boyd chaired the meeting on 7 November 1937; there were fifty-four people present. Boyd had noted that attendance at Department meetings had fallen. Conscious of publicity, as always, he sent invitations all around the medical school. The meetings became a focus for pathologists from all over Toronto and from more distant parts of Ontario. Throughout his time as Head, Boyd attended regularly, presented papers, and gave close attention to the presentations of his colleagues, particularly the younger ones.

Boyd's first ten years in Toronto were a continuation of life in Winnipeg. Klotz had been an excellent research worker who had disproved Noguchi's theory that yellow fever was caused by a spirochaete. He was respected and beloved by his staff and residents up until his death from leukaemia. He was openly critical of Boyd's books. Klotz had told the Toronto students that the man from Winnipeg was a charlatan. He was wrong; Boyd was a showman but no charlatan. Toronto students were soon to revere Boyd. He was now in charge of a larger department with several senior and competent people to take the load of routine hospital work off his shoulders. Boyd gave himself only nominal responsibility for diagnostic surgical pathology, which devolved on Dr. William Robinson, an excellent surgical pathologist. By having his own secretarial and technical staff, Robinson was semi-independent. Boyd, however, occasionally cut surgical specimens himself as late as 1946; one of his juniors remembers in particular his big powerful hands with the knife at the cut-up bench. He was capable in his Toronto days of providing a reasonable second opinion on histopathological slides. The medico-legal pathology was passed mainly to Robinson. Dr. Eric Linell was responsible for neuropathology; he smoked a pipe continuously and his hands were wizened from the constant exposure to formalin. Boyd had little enthusiasm for neuropathology, and when Linell was away he would have a great throw-out of specimens to the dismay of the returning Linell.

The staff included a librarian, Miss Williamson, who looked after the Banting Institute Library, two typists, Gwen Boyd (no relation) and Laura McKinnon, and two histotechnologists. Laura McKinnon acted as the curator of the pathological museum, safeguarding the specimens as a hen her chicks. Any specimen removed from the Museum was promptly returned to it — or else!

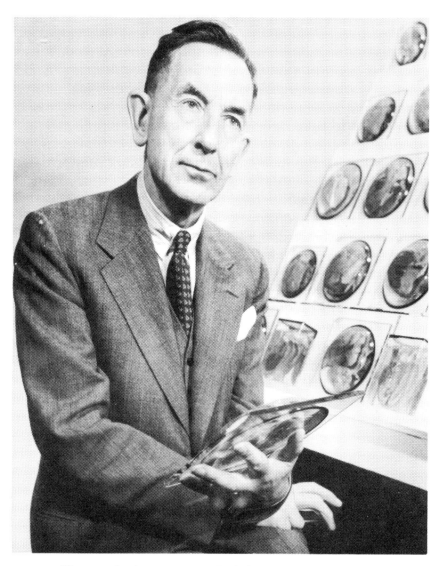

The man in the museum — Pathology Museum, Toronto

The Department of Pathology and Bacteriology occupied the first two floors of the five-storey Banting Institute, which was less than a decade old; pathology was on the main floor, with the museum in the basement. The east wing lecture theatre held 200 students, and the pathology and bacteriology laboratory on the first floor held 150 students. The building is still in use for the same purposes, a typical 1930s academic building, with an interior of dark wood, and cold corridors with stone floors, now tiled.

It was a larger department than in Winnipeg. There were three professors of pathology and one of bacteriology, twenty-three academic staff in all, including six residents and a neuropathology resident, and up to eight fellows who were often trainee clinicians.

The autopsies came from the Toronto General Hospital by the tunnel beneath College Street. They were done by junior staff under Boyd's supervision. The autopsy service was well run. The mortuary attendant, a man named Hunt, kept the heavy brass hinges on the doors of the body-storage cabinets shining like gold. But post mortems were sometimes done without gloves, and tubercle bacilli could be cultured from the floor. Reports were dictated on to wax cylinders. The junior staff presented the results of their post mortem studies and discussed them with Boyd in conference daily. They learned from him the value of the autopsy in medicine and how to present findings at meetings in coherent, organized and audible form.

Post mortems were reviewed every morning at nine. The staff sat on tiered benches over the autopsy table while microscope sections were projected by the light of a sputtering carbon arc. Some residents never learned how to operate the projector; whispers of advice from the others did little to help as Boyd, having been working already for four hours, yawned his way through the interruption. Many ex-servicemen residents, keen to be on a training ladder, chose Boyd as a good role model; he was successful, well thought of, and he attracted clinicians to his rounds. Residents learned the art of public speaking, how to make sure that the projector and flashlight pointer were working, not to overload a talk with slides, to hold the wooden pointer in the right hand and always to speak facing the audience. Simple lessons, but lessons which many fail to learn. On Wednesday mornings Boyd presided at clinico-pathological rounds attended by the whole medical staff of the hospital — many, like the Professor of Medicine, Duncan Graham, who represented the previous

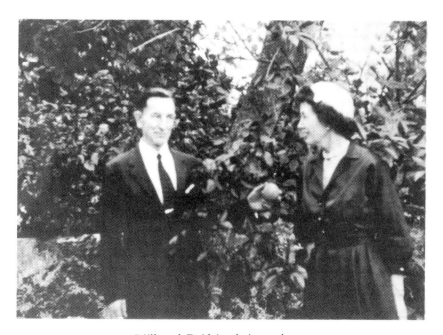
Will and Enid in their garden

generation, practised medicine based on complete physical examination of the patient. There were occasional personal tensions in the air, left over from the period of the discovery of insulin. Best did not usually attend rounds. When he was invited on one occasion, he came — to discuss a case of diabetes with renal complications. He did not in fact discuss the case, but gave a potted account of the discovery of insulin and how the physicians present had failed to make the best of a great biochemical discovery.

Boyd was by this time very much the professor, dapper in a blue suit, though sometimes quite frayed. He was conscious of his status. "My name is Dr. Boyd and I am Chief of Pathology." In the secretary's office at four o'clock over a cup of tea, he would lay down the law — graciously, but everyone knew it was being laid down. There was some initial question as to whether the residents should rise when Boyd came into the room, but the idea was tactfully quashed by one of the younger staff. On reflection Boyd thought that it was not necessary.

He was critical, convivial and popular, and had easy but sometimes superficial sympathies. The smooth Scottish voice would express concern over some personal or domestic problem of a colleague, but it would not always be quite clear how great the concern was. He had considerable personal administrative power, and sometimes used it in odd ways; for instance, there was a shortage of lily bulbs in Toronto during the war, and one garden shop opened at seven o'clock in the morning to offer one bulb to each customer. Boyd organized a long line of employees from his department, cleaners and all, each to collect one bulb, all for Boyd's garden.

Most of Boyd's time as professor in Toronto was spent against a backdrop of war—the prelude, the actuality, and the aftermath. The peaceful life of a Toronto medical professor was modified by blackouts, by extra work caused by colleagues absent on war service. Toronto boys and girls were drowned coming home on the *Athenia*, sunk forty-eight hours after Hitler had attacked Poland. Men from all over the Commonwealth came to Canada for air combat training. Salvage drives were frequent and saboteurs were suspected in factories and public utilities. Food was rationed, although stay-at-home Canadians suffered less than most.

The casualty lists were long, and families listened anxiously to the ten o'clock news, parents and grandparents stunned by what seemed to be developing into the carnage of twenty-five years earlier. Many young

Canadians died on the beach at Dieppe, in bombing raids over Germany, in Normandy and at Monte Cassino which was scarcely the "soft underbelly of Europe" as Churchill had called it. Throughout the war, Canadian corvettes protected the convoys in the North Atlantic, but the casualties amongst Canadian merchant seamen and Royal Canadian Navy crews were great. A major military hospital was founded on the grounds of Sunnybrook Farm, which had been one of the city's best afternoon walks.

Teaching and The Museum

War or no war the teaching of pathology went on unimpaired. The pathology course was traditional; 360 hours in fourth year, sixty in fifth year and sixty in sixth year, with separate pathology examinations in fourth and fifth years. It was modified in 1946 to bring pathology into the second year, but the course was essentially the same when Boyd retired as it had been when he arrived. His presence led to much more emphasis on teaching by the clinico-pathologic conference, at which he excelled. Toronto students considered pathology one of the best courses in their curriculum.

He lectured to a large class, and reorganized the teaching museum after his own familiar style. Before his arrival it was a rather dull collection of bottled specimens, to which Boyd added colour in the shape of clinical stories and background. The Toronto museum is still there in something like its original form for teaching.

Boyd's view on the importance of the museum in teaching medicine may be best understood from his own words which appeared in a late article, "The Medical Museum", a recapitulation of views stated earlier on several occasions.

> It should be superfluous to debate the teaching value of a medical museum. It is not so much what the visitor views, as what he takes away with him. Schools provide information; museums provide experience. The museum has become the only place where the separate parts into which medicine has fallen are put together again.
>
> But the specimen must be accompanied by the clinical history, and preferably by the microscopic appearance. It is not only the what that matters, but also the how and the why. What relation

has the specimen to the patient's illness? In the museum you are looking at the patient with a magic eye which gives you the answer to the what, and possibly to the how and the why....

The aim has been to make a clinico-pathological museum a place depicting disease in all its aspects. This is done by displaying, in addition to the gross specimens, illustrations of clinical conditions, microscopic appearances, x-ray findings, temperature charts, blood pictures, and so on.

In recent years the medical museum has been going out of fashion, being replaced by colour lantern slides flashed on the screen for a few seconds and never seen again. I hope I have persuaded you that such brief flashes can never replace the permanent visual record of the ravages of disease.

The handwritten dedication on a reprint of this paper in his own files is characteristic of his life-long relation to Enid. "To the best girl who has helped me with this work. William Boyd."

Organization Man
Boyd, now at the height of his powers, was still sufficiently in contact with diagnostic pathology to have some claim to be a pathologist. He enjoyed Toronto and its bustle and big-city atmosphere, and was deeply involved in the Academy of Medicine, a congenial and collegial haven of medical academe. Once a month there were crowded meetings in the small room at the Toronto Academy of Medicine. Dinner jackets were worn and Boyd kept an eye on attendance, and would enquire later of the absent residents why it was inconvenient for them to attend. He served on the Academy council, addressed it, gave generously of his time and money, and was ultimately its President.

Boyd played his part in the affairs of his specialty within the province as a charter member of the Ontario Association of Pathologists, a member of council (1940-43) and President (1943-44). In 1951 he was elected a life member. Every year between 1940 and 1948 he gave talks on a wide variety of pathological subjects. His interests were wide rather than deep in keeping with his life-long commitment to teaching the principles of pathology and their application to the practice of medicine. He gave a last talk in 1962.

From 1938, many of his speaking engagements dealt with cancer. He was in a position to exert a considerable effect on medical matters at a national level; he was a powerful force in the creation of The Canadian Cancer Society. He became Chairman of the Committee of the Canadian Medical Association which started a professional educational campaign against cancer. He was a potent member of the authorship committee which in 1938 produced the *Handbook on Cancer*, to be distributed to every Canadian doctor. He spoke about cancer on the radio and, after a conference in Ottawa on the subject, Boyd had discussions with the Minister of Health which significantly influenced the formation of the government-sponsored National Cancer Institute. Shortly afterwards, in 1948, the Minister of Health allocated three and a half million dollars to support and maintain provincial cancer programmes.

Boyd was less involved in student life than he had been in Winnipeg, but he found time to address the Medical Students' Arts and Letters Club in the 1942-43 session on his favourite topic, "Why people climb mountains". The text of this lecture makes it clear that he had a considerable knowledge of winter climbing; he had scaled the Schreckhorn, the Matterhorn, and the Grepon at Chamonix. To give a reason for mountain climbing, he quoted A.F. Mummery. "He (the mountaineer) gains a knowledge of himself, a love of all that is most beautiful in nature, and an outlet that no other sport affords for the stirring energies of youth; gains for which no price is perhaps too high." In 1948 he read and discussed "The Miracle of Purun Bhagat" by Kipling before the same group. During the war Boyd gave considerable help to Norwegian students studying in Toronto; this was recognized by an honorary doctorate from the University of Oslo in 1946.

The department gave a summer course of post-graduate lectures for aspirants to Fellowship of the Royal College of Physicians and Surgeons. Boyd always tried hard, and sometimes in vain, to find histological slides easy enough for these non-pathologists to identify. He was a kindly mentor and examiner.

He worked as hard during his Toronto days as before. Rising at 5:00 am, he wrote for two hours or more, made his breakfast, and was in the department in time to attend the daily autopsy round at 9:00 am. Weekly formal rounds were at noon. When asked by a student writer how he ordered his life so as to be so successful, Boyd replied that he usually worked on his books from 5:00 am till 8:00 am and then spent all day at work in the department. In the evenings he frequently had meetings, or attended social events; at 11:00 pm he would say his goodbyes, except perhaps at a dance, when he was often one of the last to leave, dragged away by Enid. He recommended working in short shifts at any one thing, and revealed his habit of noting on the back flyleaf important pages in a book he was reading.

Although he had little interest in forensic pathology he once acted as medical adjudicator in a hearing in an assize court relating to personal injury. Two years later he gave evidence in an inquiry under the Workmen's Compensation Act, testifying that the incidence of lung cancer in the Consumers Gas Company plant outside Toronto was six times higher than in the rest of the community.

He was no research worker and did not train juniors in experimental pathology; there was less need for this since the department was next door to the Banting and Best research building. But he was effective on committees and ran a meeting well. He was active on faculty committees, notably the library committee, and got on well with most colleagues. He was dedicated to his teaching. His lectures were virtuoso performances, as were his clinico-pathologic rounds. He was a great showman; his annual Christmas lecture to all the students and staff was to read *The Elephant Man*, a moving account of neurofibromatosis. In the winter of 1944 Toronto had a very heavy snowstorm when twenty-four inches fell overnight. The University classes were cancelled, but Boyd appeared (another professor had skiied to the campus) and gave a normal class to the half dozen students who came.

Revising the Books
The books were a constant pre-occupation. A former colleague recalled "Boyd's folder: it played a dominant feature of our lives. In fact we were its willing slaves. The whole department and all our activities were designed to feed it. 'That's a very interesting article,' Boyd would murmur. 'Would you give me your precis of it, as I will soon be starting to revise the textbook'."

> With four books needing constant revision, we were like birds feeding ravenous fledglings in the nest. Gwen Boyd and Laura McKinnon were kept busy hammering on their typewriters. It would not have occurred to Boyd to have his typing done com-

mercially. By the time Boyd sat down to the actual revision, a manila folder corresponding to each chapter would be full of references and abstracts, and at five in the morning these would be woven together in narrative form in Boyd's handwriting. Very few alterations of the initial manuscript were necessary because Boyd's saturation with good prose in his early years had left him with a clear readable style. His rules for punctuation were simple: 'The comma is only to be put in to make the meaning clear.' Only one resident ever expressed criticism of having to work for the books, for the exercise was regarded as part of training and indeed gave a sense of purpose.

The Education of a Doctor
His views on medical education were now mature. He stated them in his inaugural address as President of the Toronto Academy of Medicine, "The Education of a Doctor".

> In medical education we are standing at a crossroads, just as we are in politics and economics. Throughout the ages nearly all the fundamental changes in education have come about not as the result of inspiration from the teachers, but as pressure from the taught. The schoolmaster has not been the reformer but the reformed.

> For the last hundred years and more the chief change which the curriculum has undergone is that it has become fuller and fuller and heavier and heavier. Every year something has been added and little or nothing has been removed. Even in a subject such as anatomy, the oldest of the basic pre-clinical sciences, during the last 30 years there has been a 40 percent increase in the size of Cunningham's *Manual of Dissection*. Is it small wonder that at the end of the present-day course a considerable number of our students are intellectually stunned? They are bulging with facts which they have memorized, but their imagination, their originality and their initiative have suffered in consequence. They have been stuffed with canned food for the mind and are suffering from fatty degeneration of the intellect. It is difficult for the teacher to realize this, because it is always hard to get the view-

point of someone in a different circle. Sometimes watching from my study window a robin hopping over the lawn and picking up worms, I think "What a charming picture", but no doubt the worm thinks otherwise. Thus does the viewpoint influence our entire outlook. Truth is not absolute; it does not remain the same tomorrow as it is today. That statement could not be better illustrated than by present-day medicine. Such being the case, it is our duty to educate the minds of our young men, not only fill them with facts.

I do not believe that this can be done by means of lectures or textbooks. The most effective instrument is the question-and-answer method made famous by Socrates, provided that the questions are framed with the object of making the student's mind work, not merely pressing a button in his memory mechanism. This is best done in small groups, but it can be done even when the teacher is handicapped by a huge class. . . .

The dead hand of tradition lies heavy on the medical curriculum. For many years in Winnipeg I taught my students in the way in which I had been taught. I can still hear the sound of the pencils as every man stippled the granules of the polymorphonuclear leucocytes, a soul-deadening occupation completely devoid of educational value. The object of these long hours of microscopic study appeared to be to turn the student into a pathologist qualified to recognize the rarest tumour and to illustrate it by drawings. By slow degrees I have changed my viewpoint, have supplemented microscopic examination by the study of gross material, and have replaced the making of drawings by question and answer on sections projected on a screen and on photomicrographs in colour. The object of microscopic study by the undergraduate student should be the understanding of the disease process rather than the recognition of a given lesion. It is the destruction of the elastic tissue in the aorta by the spirochaeta pallidum that matters, not the spotting of syphilitic aortitis from the presence of perivascular collars of lymphocytes and plasma cells. At the same time I expect the future practitioner and surgeon to recognize the naked-eye appearance of carcinoma of the breast, a caseous lymph node, and diverticulitis of the colon.

He was noted as an after-dinner speaker and many of his occasional and unpublished writings date from this time. They include speeches relating to the mountains, to great writers and to matters of professional interest of the day. Immersed as he was in Toronto, he did not forget the first two universities with which he had been associated. In a speech in response to a toast to the University of Toronto he reminisced:

> I have been connected in my time with three universities, each one entirely different from the others.
>
> The first was in a grey city in Scotland where the East wind blows in the mist from the North Sea, and the rain squalls beat, and the old castle looks down on the stream of young life, and the church bells clash on a Sunday morning, a city of which Robert Louis Stevenson living in exile in the South Seas cried: "There are no stars to me like the street lamps of Edinburgh."
>
> The second was a new school, in a new city, set in the gateway to the West, where the sun burns you in summer, and the north wind freezes you in winter; but on spring nights you can hear the mournful cry of the wild geese as they fly overhead in the darkness winging their way to the Arctic, and you get the thrill of feeling that you are living on the edge of great wide spaces.

He jealously guarded the manuscripts of his talks, since he would give them repeatedly, modified only slightly to fit another audience. They were almost always a success and he would return to the Department in very good humour having done what he did best. Only once, a colleague recalls, did he come back disconcerted. The evening, a graduation talk at another Canadian university, was a drunken disaster ending in a bun fight, and nobody listened.

At Home
Soon after he arrived in Toronto he was living at "The Coolins" on Bayview Avenue — a typical, comfortable, middle-class house distinguished by its wealth of books and by the high quality of the rugs. Enid would not have a vacuum cleaner in the house and the rugs became

threadbare. The name of the house bespoke the familiar Scottish nostalgia for the hills. Enid led an active social life, playing golf and badminton. The domestic chores were looked after by a housekeeper who came in several times a week. Despite—or perhaps because of—their childlessness, Enid was ever attentive to her husband and never seemed jealous of the books which consumed so much of his life. Perhaps she realized they were his children. Their friends and his pupils all regarded them as an unusually happy couple.

He ran a journal club in his house over beer and Beethoven, at which residents and Fellows from the hospital, sometimes in dinner jackets, would present summaries of their reading. Each resident was allotted a journal and had to make a critical analysis of its contents. Boyd would pick up the summaries and put them in his folder. Later he digested the information and used it for parts of the edition he was revising at the time. Enid was in the background as a gracious hostess. Hospitality demanded its return; during the war whisky was rationed to one bottle per person per month. Junior staff were firmly requested to hand over their quota to the Professor.

His workroom, tidy to the end, had innumerable little wooden dockets into which he would stuff cards bearing information in his neat handwriting. Here the books were edited and re-edited, a constant labour. His library had big leather-bound classics: Churchill, T.E. Lawrence, Dickens, speeches. He still read widely outside medicine but used the Commonplace Book no more. Its last and only entry in his Toronto period was Landor's famous verse:

"I warmed both hands before the fire of life;
It sinks and I am ready to depart."

In the big city he turned more and more to his garden, writing on 11 July 1946, "To me a garden becomes more and more essential for the peace and happiness of the soul, for there one finds tranquillity." In earlier days he had cut flowers in the house until late October and would take them to friends in hospital. He would give his colleagues advice on their gardens, whether or not they asked for it. He grew lilies and roses, and was once seen waist deep in a three-foot pit filling it with compost. In his last ten years he never picked the flowers and never gave them away. In extreme old age he had professional gardening assistance and even gave up cutting the lawn.

Exercise sporadically taken, varied in nature from time to time. His real passion was for the mountains, but as the years passed he escaped there less often. Instead, there was golf at the Rosedale Golf Club, badminton, bridge and the Toronto Skating Club. He did not always persist in the pastimes he dallied with.

One senior physician remembers strolling with him in the hills at the Canadian Medical Association meeting in Banff soon after the end of the war:

> He smoked cigarettes which in that day and age almost everybody did; and it was not seen as a major health hazard or a character defect as it is today. He smoked a lot of them. As a semi-bankrupt medical student smoking cigarettes was out of the question for me; it was a privilege reserved for the very rich. The other thing I recall is that as we walked, talking about the countryside and the view and the beautiful weather, from time to time he picked flowers that were growing alongside the path or in the shrubbery near the path. He went to some length to pick these and then describe them by name, both common and Latin, indicating where they might be found in Scotland and other parts of the world, what drugs could be obtained from some of them and which were poisonous. . . . He was a gentle and very knowledgeable man with a beautiful way of teaching and talking.

He had a good hi-fi record player to indulge his love of music. He savoured music rather than having a profound knowledge of it. Beethoven's violin concerto was a favourite. He would take the needle off at the end of the first movement of a piano concerto and move to the third. He said he was bewitched by the sound.

He was something of a Lothario, at least in his imagination, and he enjoyed flirting and dancing with his partner held close. He unashamedly admitted, "I like to go to the meetings and kiss all the pretty girls." The puritan in him had now relaxed sufficiently to be able to quote in a speech to the ladies S.J. Perelman's quip which he had picked up from a neurosurgical colleague: "She found herself a goddess in a world controlled by gods, So she opened up her bodice and evened up the odds."

His close friends included Grant and his wife, with whom he enjoyed convivial evenings, but his wider social life was closely tied to professional obligations. As he aged he became even fonder of Scotch whisky and had a somewhat low tolerance. On convivial occasions his gait would rather easily become a little unsteady.

Curiously, for a widely read and thoughtful man, he rarely discussed politics; there is only one reference in his papers to momentous events of 1939: "Sick about the war news (Russia attacking Poland — September 17 1939)."

The Photograph and the Shaving Mirror
Life, serene and satisfying as it had been for many years, was interrupted in the early summer of 1947, by a photograph. He had been away at a meeting where someone had taken a casual photograph of him and had sent him a copy with the comment, "You seem to have a parotid tumour." A glancing shadow has thrown the small tumour into relief; when he looked for it, it was clearly visible in his shaving mirror.

The tumour, a mucous adenocarcinoma, was promptly removed by the Professor of Surgery, Robert Janes, in the Toronto General Hospital. He was left with a complete left facial palsy which later improved, but did not disappear entirely. The tumour recurred in his neck as a small nodule in December 1965, and was treated by electron-beam irradiation. He was followed up for the rest of his life at the Princess Margaret Hospital. The tumour recurred several times in his neck, on the last occasion when he was 91 years old. He wrote immediately after his first operation:

> I was extremely fortunate in getting my surgeon to let me out on the third day after operation, which was not bad, seeing that it was a three-hour job. Dr. Janes might not have allowed me to go if he had known that I cut the back lawn and sprayed it with 2-4D the day after I got home.

> The healing process has not been as comfortable as it might have otherwise been, because much of the time of the surgeon was taken up with dissecting out the branches of the facial nerve and some of these are just beginning to recover their sensibility. [*Here his anatomy was not quite right.*] This process usually is at its height between 2 & 3 am. Somebody should devote a piece of research to determining why unpleasant things connected with health usually occur at night.

But I have certainly nothing to grumble about. I had a delightfully lazy life, having breakfast on the back patio in my dressing gown, doing just as much or as little as I want to in the garden, reading all sorts of nice things and listening to lovely music. And I am even beginning to enjoy a good meal, because it is at last possible for me to open my mouth wider than a quarter of an inch.

In a few days I shall probably be starting a course of radium treatment, as the lesion proved to be malignant . . . an adenocarcinoma of the parotid, which is a really rare bird.

His colleagues in pathology, having noted in the autopsy room several unfortunate end-results of radiotherapy, persuaded him to go to Manchester; the well-known radiotherapist Ralston Paterson had recently been a visiting professor in Toronto.

He was treated by radiotherapy at the Christie Hospital and Holt Radium Institute in Manchester, then as now, one of the world's leading centres. There the nature of the tumour was reviewed and found to be a "mixed adenoid and epidermoid carcinoma". On 18 July 1948 Paterson implanted radium needles for six days, after which Boyd was discharged. Both room costs and professional fees were waived as a courtesy. Many years later Paterson recalled how after his radiotherapy, but while still in hospital, Boyd donned a white coat and went on a ward round with him.

Boyd was resilient. He wrote from the Cadogan Hotel in London a little over a month after his radiotherapy:

Life with us is extremely pleasant, and we are really having a marvellous time. The worst of the radium reaction was at Glenshee, where there was nobody to wonder at my ugly face except the sheep and the Highland cattle. The hills and the glens were as grand as ever, and the pervading peace of the place was good both for my face and my soul. The very name of Glenshee was right; it means the Glen of Peace. Then to Edinburgh for two days where I mingled with the great ones such as professors and heads of departments, people whom I used to regard with reverent awe in my student days!

> The face is behaving very well, it is hardly paining me at all, the colour is slowly returning to normal, power is coming back to the facial nerve and when you see me next I hope to be semi-presentable.

It all settled down, although it left a distortion of the handsome face; it gradually subsided, leaving only a slight flattening on the one side. When he returned to Toronto, it was straight back to work. "Sympathy is wasted on me — book me for my full schedule of lectures." He was usually thereafter photographed in profile or half profile, as the famous photograph by Karsh shows. His cancer left him alone for nearly sixteen years; and for the next five years in Toronto he taught and wrote with but little diminished vigour. He had a special interest in the microscopic slides of his tumour and used a photomicrograph of it as an illustration in one of his texts.

There was nothing new in his professional life after this point — a remaking of the same speeches and a re-editing of the same books. The tide of life usually reaches the high-water mark by sixty, ebbing slowly thereafter. Boyd's tide ebbed more slowly than most, but by now he had drifted from the practice of pathology, blown by the winds of writing and to a lesser degree by the duties of administration. "In his latter days he knew little pathology, and had no focussed grasp of the difficult areas. Research — he had no mind for it." So said a close friend. Still lecturing and writing marvellously well, he was creating his own myth, and more and more was to live within it.

In 1950, when he was set to retire, he happily accepted the university's offer of another year's employment. He gave his last paper to a departmental meeting on 7 May 1951, on the pathology of the ground substance of the mesenchyme, more grist for the ever ready mills of the next edition.

When he left in 1951, the Pathology Museum, so long the focus of his attention, was named in his honour, and the library of the Toronto Academy of Medicine was similarly designated. Plaques were unveiled in both places. The Academy (the museum and library have now moved to the Toronto General Hospital) exhibited a bronze statuette of him — sitting as in a showcase surrounded by memorabilia, and nearby his unpublished writings and manuscripts. On top of his papers sat his ice-axe, mute witness of days in the Coolins long ago.

---- Chapter 10 ----

Evening

EVENING HAD drawn on. Men become old when they believe inwardly and privately in their own personal mortality, a revelation that can come surprisingly late even to pathologists, close as they are to the paraphernalia of death. Boyd's first retirement was in 1951 when he was sixty-six. It was only the very beginning of his old age.

Vancouver in 1951 was not yet a glittering metropolis, but a medium-sized port city just over sixty-five years old. It depended for its prosperity on trade, local agriculture, horticulture and forestry. The Art Deco City Hall, built in 1936, was an early phase in the construction of a high-rise city centre, but World War II slowed development. Park Royal, Canada's second major shopping centre, had been opened in West Vancouver in 1950. The gardens flourished and blossomed in the mild wet climate, and the style of life in the wooden houses in the spreading suburbs was a pleasant compromise between Canadian and Californian. The University of British Columbia had been founded in 1908 in beautiful parkland at the edge of the city overlooking the sea; its medical school was new, founded after many years of hesitation.

Boyd's appointment as foundation professor of pathology was fortunate for him and for the university. The university obtained a man of world renown in his profession to start off the department and, in the event, to aid in the maturation of the young but highly competent local pathologists. By now an experienced and wily university administrator, he was given a new lease on life and a base from which to travel over North America, and sometimes further. He was now more than an invited lecturer; he was a cult figure. The day of the single-author text was coming to a close, but a single author who could write well could still produce a sufficient semblance of authenticity to suffice.

The correspondence between the Dean (Dr. Myron Weaver) and Boyd indicates that the University was keen to hire him. Boyd wrote that he was receiving $9000 from the University of Toronto, plus $1000 from the Toronto General Hospital, and that a ten percent increase was due, adding that his major equipment request was an epidiascope and projector for gross material. The prompt reply was that the University of British Columbia and the Vancouver General Hospital between them were prepared to find $12,000. Boyd also asked for plenty of help with teaching — to ensure that he had time left for his beloved books.

An additional inducement was that the provincial legislature had just voted $750,000, a fair sum in the early 1950s, to provide a new building in which pathology, among other medical sciences, would be housed. Boyd wanted a title such as "Senior Professor" or "Distinguished Professor", but the Senate was not willing to grant his request, and Boyd had to be content to be the Professor and Head, and on annual re-appointment to conform to the policy of the university for the appointment of staff over sixty-five.

Founding Academic Pathology

The first meeting of the University of British Columbia Faculty of Medicine was on Thursday, 12 October 1950. Shortly afterwards Boyd began assiduously to attend the meetings. He was clearly able to establish his subject firmly in the curriculum; it was taught in the 2nd, 3rd and 4th years, and heavily weighted in the 2nd year.

When Boyd arrived, there were six pathologic anatomists in the three major hospitals in the Vancouver area, two at the Vancouver General Hospital, two at St. Paul's and two at the Royal Columbia Hospital in New Westminster. They all had cross-appointment to the Faculty of Medicine. The large autopsy service at the Vancouver General Hospital carried out over 1200 autopsies a year at that time, so there was a good source of teaching material. The basic science departments of the faculty,

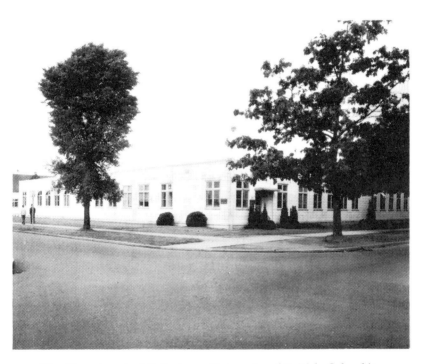

The Department of Pathology, University of British Columbia, early 1950s

including pathology, were housed in temporary war-time huts on the campus some eight miles from the Vancouver General Hospital. Boyd had a small area in one of the huts which included his office, a small office for a teaching fellow, a laboratory for one technician to prepare histologic slides, and another room which he promptly turned into a museum. The arrangement was adequate for the teaching of general pathology, but to teach special pathology, tissues had to be transported to the campus from the hospitals in garbage bags for use in the practical classes.

He brought with him from Toronto some of his own teaching material and set about organizing a pathology course with the enthusiastic co-operation of the younger Vancouver pathologists. His teaching philosophy would not be out of place even in 1992: "The best way to learn to think about a subject is to have to answer questions. Instead of being taught pathology, it is much better to be taught how to learn pathology, although this is much more difficult for the teacher."

He had overall responsibility for pathology in the Vancouver General Hospital and for the planning of its new Pathology Department there, and took the early steps towards co-operation with St. Paul's Hospital and the Shaughnessy Hospital, steps essential in building up an integrated community of pathologists within the city. This community, one of his successors believes, flourishes to this day. While his energy and ability were clearly outstanding for his age, the drive was now flagging a little.

Boyd's own collection of teaching slides was supplemented by both gross and microscopic material from the Vancouver General Hospital. He regularly attended autopsy demonstrations, seminars and conferences at the hospital, obtaining teaching material and contributing to the seminars. He also attended clinical, medical and surgical conferences to keep abreast of advances in the practice of medicine. His colleagues soon found out that, even if no longer a "practical pathologist", as a teacher he was without parallel. He attended the meetings of the British Columbia Association of Pathologists and the Pacific North West Association of Pathologists, and was a popular speaker at American meetings. He now revelled in his own legend, telling tales of his earlier days — how he had been popular at meetings of American pathologists during prohibition days because he always carried two bottles of Scotch with him.

Vancouver was smaller and less sophisticated than Toronto, but Boyd fitted well into the academic medical scene. He lived at 5916 North West

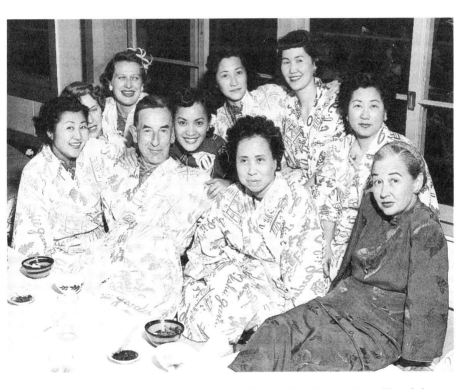

Rejuvenescence: speaker at American Cancer Society meeting, Honolulu 1951

Marine Drive, a house with a pleasant garden about a mile from campus, where the Toronto pattern of musical evenings with hospitality for staff and at least some students was repeated. He was still popular with students and fitted into the Vancouver medical establishment well. Acquaintances of that time remember the dapper figure, usually in a three-piece suit, the life and soul of any party, talking, always talking, usually with a glass in his hand. He was at times a magnificent party performer, falling on his knees before the ladies and declaiming from "Romeo and Juliet". Enid was patient and tolerant towards his clowning. She had herself grown out of the youthful exuberance that her husband still obviously enjoyed; but if his antics embarrassed her she disguised her feelings beneath a radiant smile. She was indeed the epitome of the gracious professor's wife, supportive of her husband even to the suppression of her own inclinations, and unfailingly kind and hospitable to students and junior staff.

His wit still twinkled against the hint of the puritan background. In a lecture to the British Columbia Division of the Canadian Cancer Society in Vancouver he quipped, "A preacher always preaches best under a sense of sin. A course in practical sin might be recommended in his training. Or even a half course, or for those no longer young a short refresher course." He was an honorary life member, director and past national president of the society. As in Toronto, the medical school held him in high regard, a respected, almost revered father figure whose pre-Christmas lecture on the "Elephant Man" was as popular as it had been in Toronto. As in Toronto he taught by the lecture, still a spectacular performance, and by the clinico-pathologic case conference.

Those who knew him in his semi-retired Vancouver days remember him as no longer a skilled diagnostic pathologist, indeed almost a dilettante, but still a potent political figure in the medical school. He and others were pressing hard for a new medical school building in which pathology would be more amply accommodated.

He was generous in many large things, but parsimonious in small ones. He would boast, after having been someone's guest for a weekend, that he had not spent a dime.

His museum Fellow was Dr. Clarisse (Lore) Aszkanazy (later Dolman), a 1947 graduate of the University of Toronto. Like many men of his time, Boyd had an aversion to women in a professional role; but Lore was an exception to the general rule. Despite the gap of years between them, she and Enid became firm friends. The museum which Boyd started with her help in Vancouver was modelled on that in Toronto and has now, after his death, grown into something that would have met with his approval.

Even before he came to Vancouver he had spent much time in travelling, in response to invitations mainly from universities. This continued during his Vancouver years as, more than ever, his lecturing skills were in demand. He was sometimes away for months at a time. The requests to the Dean for leave become more frequent, finally culminating in a "conversation" with the Dean, and a letter to Boyd, in which the Dean received his resignation "regretfully". The detail of the conversation remains unknown. The time for retiring had clearly come, even to Boyd at last. Dean Weaver in valediction at a faculty meeting on 11 May 1954 accurately referred to him as "the outstanding teacher of pathology of our generation".

To Mature Like Old Wine
He could now return "to mature like old wine among his friends" in his beloved Toronto. He missed the maturity and urbanity of Toronto, and particularly its Academy of Medicine. He had made many friends in Vancouver and was invited back for several consecutive years to give some historical lectures as well as lectures in pathology. By this time he was well into his seventies but he still cast his spell over his young and critical audiences.

He visited his old department in Toronto regularly but by 1960, as one of his successors recalls, whatever he had bequeathed to pathology at the University of Toronto had largely vanished. He still attended teaching sessions with students and residents but was more concerned with the quality of presentation than with the material presented. His excessive demands on secretarial help, offered as a courtesy to him by the active staff, caused some annoyance to his successors and tarnished his image among those in the department who had to put up with him. In spite of his tactlessness he was welcomed at seminars in Sunnybrook Hospital until late in life.

Alabama Winters
It was Alabama, however, which gave him the opportunity to escape from Toronto winters. The distinguished American pathologist J.F.A.

McManus invited Boyd for several winters to the University of Alabama, where he did a little teaching, advised on the modification of the museum, and clearly gave much pleasure to students and younger colleagues. Now over seventy years old, he still gave good value for money.

Of Boyd in his later years, McManus recalls:

> His voice was a remarkable instrument that could produce emphases and indicate nuances of meaning that his entranced audiences rarely failed to understand. His delivery lost nothing from the remnants of his native Scottish brogue he retained, positive but not obtrusive to the point of interfering with the understanding and appreciation of his words.
>
> At the beginning of a talk, Boyd would place himself and his notes at the rostrum carefully, clear his throat, and give the customary acknowledgements to the group and its officers, and to any other dignitaries. After an appreciable pause, Dr. Boyd would take the audience's attention by some jocular reference or allusion to his hosts or to the meeting, to the geography or what not, or by some self-deprecatory comment. . . . The presentation was effortless and apparently unrehearsed, but much thought and attention had gone into it. . . . He studied and refined the details of presentation. Boyd distinguished between the paper for publication and the same material presented verbally, the latter to be compressed and "ruthlessly expurgated", removing all irrelevant detail. Most important, Boyd castigated the speaker who did not address his audience.
>
> It was not a native ability.
>
> When he decided to become a teacher, and realized that public speaking would be required of him, the young medical student decided that the Edinburgh University Union, the student debating group, was where he could and should gain the experience he required. Dr. Boyd said he was so shy that several visits were made to the Union meetings with every intention to speak, before he mustered up the courage to do so. These were the beginnings of one of the great speakers of medicine.

McManus remembered a trip with Boyd through rural Alabama, "by car along two-lane roads with heavy traffic in parts, through worked-out

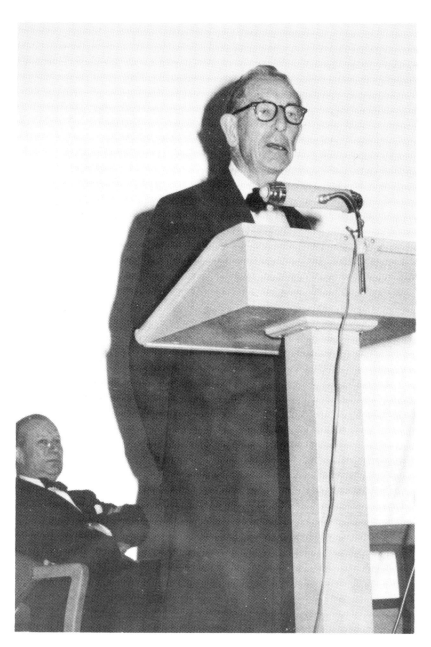

Boyd lecturing in the University of Manitoba, when over 80 years old

cotton land and red gumbo fields with empty tenant farm houses."

> Boyd saw the bland tiresome scenery with new and enthusiastic eyes, delighting in pointing out the attractive, the unusual, and the remarkable on the way. The familiar became something new and to be admired. Boyd's chief gift was a contagious enthusiasm, an ability to give new significance to the ordinary and the mundane.

McManus never forgot the letters of encouragement he received from Boyd when McManus was still a young pathologist eager to make his way.

Boyd gave major lectures as late as 1963 and was still energetic enough in 1965 to publish his last book, on the spontaneous regression of cancer. "P.S.", he wrote in 1968 at the end of a letter, "started on a new edition of the Textbook." But the years were telling and in the same year at the age of eighty-three he noted, "book pressure too great". Secretarial assistance was paid for by the publisher, but he was to continue to send generous Christmas gifts to his old secretary well into retirement, and substantial donations of money to the Toronto Academy in recognition of the excellent service he had received from the library staff over many years. In 1975 his wife noted in a letter that he was "as busy as a beaver". In that year too he still held senior honorific office in the World Pathology Foundation. By 1976 he had given up the rounds of golf that he and Enid had enjoyed together for so long.

He was now an old man. His friends were dying and his own health deteriorating. A visit to Atlanta in 1970 to give a memorial lecture was spoiled by an episode of thrombophlebitis. The changes in the world of pathology did not always please him. In the Manitoba Medical School, the Boyd museum, once the heart of the teaching of pathology, had been reduced to a small room. "Think of the present set-up," he wrote with a sniff in 1973 of the teaching of pathology in Winnipeg.

The Scottish medical world was late to recognize his achievements — perhaps his books sold better than their own. He took great delight in an invitation from the Edinburgh Royal College of Surgeons to be its first Wade Professor, a distinguished visiting professorship which entailed giving lectures and demonstrations in Edinburgh. "They had to give me the Fellowship, I would never have passed the exam." His niece tells of his meeting with his old friend Archie Christie on that occasion. "Archie and Bill were great friends and both loved their booze; Archie drove Bill the wrong way down a one-way street." They enjoyed themselves in spite of their complaint that Edinburgh was expensive.

In old age the human appreciation of mortality and the human condition becomes more acute with diminishing horizons. Boyd wrote a lay sermon in his later days — the manuscript is undated, but certainly after 1945, probably much after 1945. It gives some idea of his view of the world on his maturity and old age, a view, initially Christian becoming grey, stoical, but still essentially moral after being tempered by a world war. The Free Kirk was long in the past, but the important thing about a puritan upbringing is often the sad seriousness that is left after belief fades. The sermon is not perhaps original, and probably at least partly borrowed from an uncertain source. It is hard to find in Boyd's papers evidence of that rare quality — deep original thought. The sermon is rather a distillation of the ideas of others from many sources, well phrased, honest, and likely to appeal to educated folk in the same agnostic dilemma.

A Lay Sermon—Why?

In the lives of all of us — to some often, to others but seldom — there come moments when with an overpowering rush we are overwhelmed with that tremendous question: Why? It may be a still small voice knocking at the door of the heart, or it may be a tremendous interrogation mark painted upon the sky at night, but however — whenever it comes it is apt to prove profoundly disturbing.

This everlasting question comes echoing down the ages. "The mountains look on Marathon — and Marathon looks on the sea," the eternal snows of Everest catch century by century the clear light of this morning, the calm face of the Sphinx looks out over the unchanging desert, and poor man, the atom of a day, lifts his face to the vast dome of the sky, and utters his endless cry, why, why, why?

To the ordinary man this question comes but seldom, and perhaps it is well that this is so, but come at times it will. In the gaiety and gloom of a ballroom where youth and beauty meet to chase the glowing hours with flying feet, he pauses for a moment, looks round upon this giddy throng, and suddenly that little voice whispers, "Well, what is the meaning of it all?" Man, with his burning soul, was put upon this round earth surely for some special purpose. Is this mode of life, this manner of spending night after night, a fulfillment of that great purpose? And thus the voice is stilled, you glance at your programme, and go in search of your next partner. Or out upon the hills at night you lift your eyes and consider the heavens where glitter those millions of worlds at such incredible distances away, each holding its own secret, and again that tremendous question crushes you down: What is the meaning of it all? And again the mood passes, you light your pipe, and set yourself to the task of picking your way and avoiding the loose stones.

How differently has this question been answered by the children of men throughout the ages! And how simple are some of the answers. The Scottish Catechism opens with this very question: What is man's chief end? And the answer seems so simple: Man's chief end is to glorify God and enjoy him for ever. Simple, yes, but is it satisfying? How are we to glorify God, and how can we enjoy him forever? People are apt to think that this man of science, the very prototype of the enquiring questioner, may furnish us with an answer, but surely this is a vain hope which can never be realized. Science may clarify our vision, it may sweep aside the mists of ignorance and superstition, but it can never answer this question. For, indeed it is concerned with another question, not why, but how. Science can tell us how life behaves, not why it is here. It can number the stars of this firmament, it can tell us the very elements of which they are composed, but their ultimate meaning is beyond it.

Surely it is to the philosophers and the poets that we should turn for a solution of this tremendous problem. And from them we receive what is perhaps the only answer that we shall ever get, an answer which varies from complete hopelessness to seeking refuge in a mysticism which must appeal to poor mankind as long as the unanswerable remains unanswered. Dante has given us the answer of the mystic in our tremendous lives which, if we can accept it, will still all our anxious questioning. "In la sue

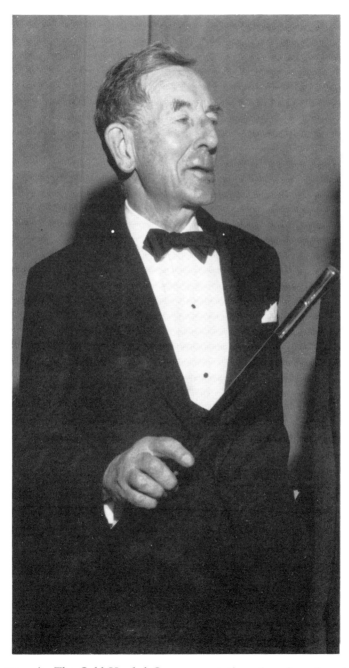

The summit. The Gold-Headed Cane presentation. American Association of Pathologists and Bacteriologists, Montreal 1962

voluntade e nostra pace." No answer of science can compete with that answer of the sad Florentine, if we can but accept it. . . . How strangely similar is our modern answer. In one of the most recent novels the hero is upon his deathbed. "He lay there thinking in an absolute mental calm, looking out upon the little ocean of his life, its currents and storms forgotten, merely pondering upon its ultimate utility. What was the good of this life? he asked. . . . He was not complaining. He had had a good time, and the world was an astonishing place, well worth a visit. But surely there was something else. Life wasn't just a museum, through which one wandered, delighted with the strange things all around one, going out finally into the night, nothing done. Surely one left something behind.

The end of the manuscript carries the pencilled note in Boyd's handwriting. "What shadows we are, and what shadows we pursue."

Pottering in a Garden
By 1960 Boyd was an old man. The allotted span was past. He could remember, in this missile age, the death of Queen Victoria. He and Enid spent their last years in 40 Arjay Crescent, Willowdale, the house in which they settled on returning from Vancouver, looked after by a devoted "help", Mildred Manning. It was a comfortable middle-class house, filled with books; the picture of Portsoy was still on his study wall beside a view of the Matterhorn. Much of his time in the summer was spent pottering in the large gardens among beds bright with roses. Christian Dior and Tropicana were among his favourites. The theatre at Stratford was one of the few distractions that would take him and Enid from their home and garden overlooking the great wooded ravine of the Don River.

Alcohol, usually Scotch, was a consolation for the passing of the years; he noted in a letter (4 November 1957), "Was in dentist's hands yesterday for two extractions — 40 minutes. Happily I was able to drink 2 glasses of rye 3 hours later — as a prophylactic against hepatitis. Roses still blooming, and still having to cut the grass." He noted in 1968, "I develop a craving for almonds and wolf them down in huge quantities, washing them down in transit with great drafts of liquor and wine."

He kept up a regular correspondence with his friends in Winnipeg, including Lennox Bell, who had become Dean of Medicine, and with the

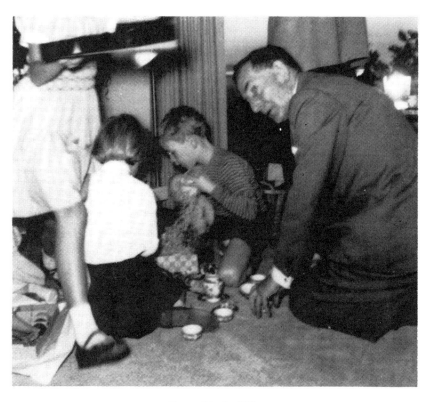

Great Uncle Billy

Winnipeg surgeon P.H.T. Thorlakson. He still accepted invitations to lecture and still retained the slightly flat Scottish accent, the wit and the pleasure in his own success. He wrote to Thorlakson on the 12th November 1970, "The affair at Atlanta was the only occasion when I had a standing ovation at the beginning of my talk, and another at the end. It was nice that Enid was there, she came as my nurse, as the wound from the last cancer operation had not yet healed."

The books kept him busy till his early eighties, updating and checking proofs. He still received many letters from student readers, mainly in the Indian sub-continent, nearly all reverential in tone. He took great joy in answering these. He was delighted when his millionth copy was printed and went round telling all his friends. He had been comparatively wealthy for a long time; the royalties from his books were a guarantee against poverty, as well as an assurance of his own continuing significance.

Enid was always with him. Neither of them talked much of their private lives, but the public view that theirs was a life-long happy marriage was almost certainly true. "It was a very close partnership. Enid was not jealous of his books. They travelled widely together, and her happy, outgoing personality made them doubly welcome wherever they went." In a casual quotation in one of his manuscripts he wrote: "Perhaps he murmured, a little sadly, how love fled . . . and hid his face among a cloud of stars." After sixty years it did not seem that love had fled from Enid and Will.

His letters to his niece Cleone Stoloff were those of a man who still took joy in life, not least in the growing tribe of great-nephews and great-nieces. Christmas time had always meant cheques for the nieces, presents for their children, and liquor bottles for their husbands. At Christmas parties he played with the children, usually on the floor, or insisted on a performance from a ten-year-old ballet student. Dinner celebrations with friends went on well into old age. Cleone remembers how he would take time to listen and offer wise counsel in times of personal stress. His generosity was not limited to advice; it also took the more practical form of financing a trip to Europe for her daughter and herself. Her most vivid and enduring memory of him is in his slippers, in the bar of the Algonquin Hotel in New York, with more than one dram in him, declaiming poetry in his finest oratorical intonation.

His own pathology plagued him. The salivary cancer, treated in 1947,

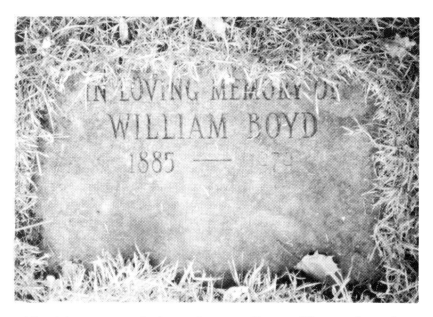

All strivings cease — St. James Cemetery, Toronto (Photograph courtesy of William Halliday)

recurred for the first of several times sixteen years later. He recorded with some pride (22 June 1966) that after seeing his cancer specialist, he cut the 4000 square feet of lawn and then left for the theatre at Stratford all on the same day. Betatron irradiation arrested the advance of the recurrence, but the skin of the ear broke down from the effect of the old and recent radiation. He reflected regretfully, "It will probably prevent the Tokyo trip." He had to decline an invitation to Vancouver in 1975 because of ill health and in 1976 he fell down the steps at Sunnybrook Hospital and broke a clavicle.

He worried about his health and treated himself in unconventional ways, taking lecithin in an attempt to slow the effects of aging. His anxiety was hardly justified since until he was over eighty he remained remarkably fit. But by 1974 he no longer heard well and suffered from an ataxia sufficiently severe to be an embarrassment at a big meeting. He had to decline an invitation to the 25th anniversary celebration of the University of British Columbia Medical School. By 1975 he wrote of failing vision and became quite blind towards the end. The stoic spirit that saw him through Flanders trenches had not left him. On 26 June 1976 he wrote, "Talking about things going well, did I tell you that I had my sixth operation for cancer two months ago? So now I have had the same cancer for 25 years and have enjoyed excellent health." The next year his femur fractured.

Old age did not defeat him entirely. He remained an impeccable dresser till late in his life. He wore beautiful ties and had a new dinner jacket tailored when in his eighties. Some of the old sparkle and a little of the Free Kirk mindset stayed till the end. Later, probably much later than 1945, musing as an unbeliever over the existence of life after death, he cut short his speculations with, "one would as soon analyze the agony of Gethsemane." He did not believe in an after life.

During his last year, and when nearly bedridden, he had several severe respiratory infections which might have released him from a life devoid of real meaning had they not been treated with antibiotics. He had fully intended to end his own life if it became untenable but in the end, to the surprise of some of his relatives, he clung to it. Pneumonia, the old man's friend finally took him. "Men must endure their going hence, even as their coming hither," he had quoted in his commonplace book. He departed this life on 10 March 1979.

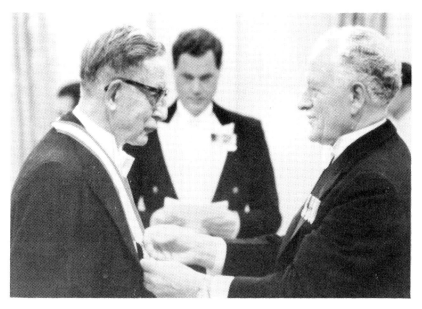

Another summit. Investiture by the Rt. Hon. Roland Michener, Governor General of Canada; Companion of the Order of Canada

The Measure of a Life
How can one see William Boyd's achievements, as he pottered in his garden? How did he recall them? The purpose of this memoir is to raise a ghost, not nail down a coffin — so the catalogue of posts, honours and invited lectures is relegated to an appendix. He particularly enjoyed the Golden Edition of the *Canadian Medical Journal*, the first issue of Volume 86, 1962, which was dedicated to him, and later his inclusion in Karsh's gallery of famous medical figures, and his appointment as a Companion of the Order of Canada. One can ask his friends. Dr. John Barrie, a close friend who smoothed his path in his latter days and helped his widow in many ways wrote:

> Over a span of 65 years he averaged one and a half articles in medical journals a year, and during the 30 years that I knew him, he averaged one major speaking engagement a month, beside giving most of the undergraduate lectures, running a busy department and setting up pathology museums all over the country. I never saw him show signs of stress, because like all professionals, he made all this look easy and had plenty of time to listen to people.

> He bore old age with fortitude. More than 60 years before he went blind, bereft of his chief joy in life, but uncomplaining, he had copied down from Milton. "There is no misery in being blind. It would be miserable not being able to bear blindness."

William Boyd's popularity as a person, writer and speaker was not difficult to analyze. As a person he was devoid of affectation, ill-nature or jealousy and thus did not inspire them in others. He had a sense of humour, but was never flippant and liked some degree of formality in his department. He was prodigal with praise and could rebuke without giving offence. When he heard or read something that appealed to him, he would often sit down and write a letter of appreciation to the author. At meetings, even if the author had paralyzed his audience with boredom, Boyd would rise slowly to his feet, clear his throat and point out something of excellence or interest that had been said. As a speaker, he had the mastery of rhythm, phrase and timing that imbues a text with greater impact than the words. In this, he brought the skills of the heart, the stage and the pulpit to the podium.

Barrie's last word was, "Faced with a difficult situation, one would have no better solution, than by saying to oneself: 'What would Boyd have done?' " Thus said a friend. Obituaries are notorious sources of whitewash, but to have friends who will write such an obituary is not entirely good luck.

The only significant professional criticism levelled against him was that he was not a great scientist. He said it himself in a letter to Bernard Weilbrenner, Acting Dominion Archivist, 27 July 1971: "I have made no original contributions to medical science." He was, however, as good a scientist as most of his critics. One man in his time can play only a limited number of parts; he should be judged on what he did, not on what he chose not to do.

What is William Boyd's place in the history of medicine? He did some competent research, all morbid anatomical. He made no contribution to experimental biological science; it was not his metier. He was a competent diagnostic histopathologist in his younger days, and spent half an ordinary professional lifetime as a conscientious practitioner. This skill like many others has to be used or lost. Like many another senior pathologist, he didn't continue to use it.

He taught and inspired medical students for sixty years, either by voice or by the printed word. And made an outstanding contribution to undergraduate medical education in pathology, by his insistence on its integration with clinical medicine and by his excellence as both lecturer and Socratic teacher. He made real contributions to the training of medical and surgical post-graduates by transmitting his skill in teaching in the autopsy room. His books carried his ideas round the medical world. He was the outstanding teacher of pathology of his generation.

He trained many successful pathologists who in their old age speak well of that training. He did little to train young men and women to be experimental pathologists of the next generation; he was not himself an experimentalist.

He held senior administrative office in University Departments of Pathology for 40 years. Pathology in Winnipeg bore his mark for many years, as his successors were his pupils, but now there is little sense that he left a significant academic legacy. In Toronto his effect was even less lasting; the discipline of pathology had formed there long before he arrived. Oblivion comes to human effort sooner than we think. The Department of Pathology at the University of British Columbia still bears some mark of his presence; and the Canadian Association of Pathologists remembers him by a Lectureship. These three medical schools and the University of Alabama all remember him by a pathology museum, of varying significance, bearing his name. In a long professional life he made many friends whose affection lingers, blossoming in the dust.

In the old man pottering in his garden lingered the ghost of a Scots boy, of a medical youth in Edinburgh, of a young doctor whose freshness was bruised but not obliterated in Flanders, of a Canadian professor whose writings were read with profit, wherever pathology was studied, of an intellectual lamplighter who lit up minds. Boyd bore the tribulations of age bravely, fortunate in his rose garden, his books and the company of his beloved wife, Enid, who survived him by six years.

"The little man," Boyd quoted, "thinks he has disposed of a great man if he can tie a label to him, as one might pin out and label a butterfly in a collection." Smaller men have tried to pin Boyd out, but he would not be pinned out readily. His greatness lay in the magic of words, used to teach young men and women how to be observant physicians. To his basic craft of pathologic diagnosis he added something enduring. He was a weaver of words, and a man remembered by his friends and students with gratitude and affection. There is no absolute measure for a life: by most reckonings William Boyd's was a good one.

Notes

Chapter 1

Several appreciations of Boyd's life have been written. These have been quoted extensively in this and other chapters.

Barrie, H.J. *Canad. Med. Assoc. J.* (1982) *126*: 421-424.

ADK (A.D. Kelly) Aequanimitas *Canad. Med. Assoc. J.* (1967) *96*: 60-61.

Feasby, W.R. *Medical Post* 16 August 1966, The Boyd Secret: hard work and gentle charm / ibid. 30 August 1966 Poetry wins a top prize in psychiatry. 13 September 1966 Edinburgh leaves its mark. / ibid. 16 August 1974 The Senior pathologist reflects on a crowded career.

McManus, J.F.A. William Boyd: A biographical sketch *Amer. J. Surg. Path.* (1979) 3: 377-381.

Anonymous Obituary *Canad. Med. Assoc. J.* (1979) 23: 1547.

A videotape of Boyd in old age gives valuable information. This is held by the Hannah Institute, Toronto.

Chapter 2

The information about Portsoy derives largely from the *Second Statistical Account of Scotland*, and from newspapers in the Portsoy Public Library, notably Anonymous: Notes on Portsoy. *Banffshire Journal* 20 September 1938.

Phillips, A. *My Uncle George: The Respectful Recollections of a Backslider in a Highland Manse.* London: Pan, 1986.

Ferguson, T. *The Dawn of Scottish Social Welfare* Glasgow: Nelson, 1947.

Youngson, A.J. *The Scientific Revolution in Victorian Medicine* London: Croom Helm, 1979.

Wohl, A.S. *Endangered Lives: Public Health in Victorian Britain* Cambridge, Mass.: Harvard University Press, 1983.

Chapter 3

The information on Edinburgh student days derives from:

Boyd, W. The Boyd Papers to be lodged in Fisher Library of University of Toronto. Where necessary, further identification is given within the text. These are quoted extensively in this and following chapters.

Boyd, W. *Cause and Effect.* The Fifth Alexander Gibson Memorial Lecture. *Canad. Med. Assoc. J.* (1965) 92: 868.

Edinburgh University Calendars 1901-1912.

Hutton, I. *Memories of a Doctor in War and Peace*. London: Heinemann, 1960.

Lechler, J.H. "Reminiscences of a Nonagenarian" *University of Edinburgh Journal* (1975) 27: 119-125.

Turner, A.L. ed. *History of the University of Edinburgh 1883-1933*. Edinburgh: Oliver & Boyd, 1933.

Turner, A.L. *Story of a Great Hospital*. The Royal Infirmary of Edinburgh 1729-1929. Edinburgh: Oliver and Boyd, 1937.

Chapter 4

The information on Derby derives from

Craven, M. *Derby. An Illustrated History*. Derby: Breedon, 1988.

The information on hospitals contained in this chapter derives from Archivists in Derbyshire, and Lancashire, and Wolverhampton Metropolitan Borough Council, Winwick Hospital (County Asylum). Dr. I. Bronks, Consultant Psychiatrist, Kingsway Hospital, Derby, and Dr. K.W.M. Scott, Consultant Pathologist, Wolverhampton Royal Infirmary.

Bowley, A.L. *Wages and Income in the United Kingdom since 1860*. Cambridge: University Press, 1937 gives information on relative incomes.

Chapter 5

The information here derives largely from Boyd, W. *With a Field Ambulance at Ypres*. The material was published in *Manitoba Medicine*, and is republished by permission of the Editor.

A good account of the early gas attacks is given in Macphail, A. *Official History of the Canadian Forces in the Great War 1914-19, The Medical Services*, pp. 290-306. Ottawa: Minister of National Defence, 1925.

More general recent studies:

Dancocks, D.G. *Welcome to Flanders Fields*. Toronto: McClelland & Stewart, 1988.

Goodspeed, D.J.K. *The Road Past Vimy: The Canadian Corps 1914-1918*. Toronto: Macmillan Canada, 1969, Toronto: General Paperbacks, 1987.

Wolff, L. *In Flanders Fields* (orig. 1958) Toronto: General Paperbacks, 1988.

Chapters 6 and 7

The information on Winnipeg derives largely from

Gray, J.H. *The Winter Years, The Depression on the Prairies*. Toronto: Macmillan, 1966.

Gutkin, H., Gutkin, M. *The Worst of Times the Best of Times*. Markham: Fitzhenry & Whiteside, 1987.

McColl, F.M. *Vignettes of Early Winnipeg 1912-1926*. Winnipeg: McColl, 1981.

Peterkin, A., Shaw, M. *Mrs. Doctor: Reminiscences of Manitoba Doctors' Wives*. Winnipeg: Prairie Publishing Co., 1976.

The information on the Medical School derives largely from the minutes of the Faculty and its executive 1910-1938, Archives of the Faculty of Medicine, University of Manitoba Medical Library. University of Manitoba Calendars 1910-1938.

University of Manitoba Medical Journal (1929-1938) 1-11.

Medovy, H. Oral history with Dr. C.G. Roland 1982. University of Manitoba Archives — courtesy of Z. Gawron.

Conversations with Dr. B. Best, Dr. J. Martin, and Dr. H. Medovy.

Dr. J. Hoogstraaten; unpublished ms history of the Department of Pathology, University of Manitoba

Chapter 8

The information on Boyd's books comes from the collection in the Manitoba authors' section in the University of Manitoba Medical Library. Random book reviews are preserved in the Boyd papers.

Chapter 9

The information on Toronto derives largely from Kilbourn W. *Toronto Remembered. A Celebration of the City*. Toronto: Stoddart Publishing, 1984.

Archives of University of Toronto, Fisher Library. Information is less freely available, being held under a fifty-year rule.

Minute book, Department of Pathology, University of Toronto, Department meetings 1921-1953 (Fisher Library, University of Toronto Archives).

Records of the Christie Hospital, Manchester.

Conversations with Drs D. Adams, M.D. Silver, A.C. Ritchie.

Boyd. W.: The Medical Museum *J.R. Coll. Surg. Edinb.* (1972) *17*: 325-328.

Boyd, W.: On the Dangers of Scrappiness *University of Manitoba Medical Journal* (1937) *8*:91-2, *Winnipeg Free Press*.

Chapter 10

Information on the University of British Columbia derives from the Archives of the Faculty of Medicine, and from conversations with Drs E.J. Bowmer, C. Dolman, D. Hardwick, H. Taylor.

The main sources in this chapter are Boyd's correspondence, the biographical articles cited, and the recollections of Cleone Stoloff.

Turnbull, F. "The curtain couldn't rise: Starting a medical school in British Columbia". *BC Medical Journal* (1987) *29*: 82-7.

Appendix 1

Curriculum Vitae
William Boyd 1885-1979

Parents   Dugald Cameron Boyd & Eliza Marion Butcher
            Married 1867 Mahableshewar, Bombay, India

Born   21 June 1885 Portsoy, Scotland

Married   2 June 1919 to Enid Christie, Winnipeg

Died   10 March 1979

Degrees and Prizes
1908	MBChB, University of Edinburgh
1911	MD, University of Edinburgh, Honours and Gold Medal
1912	Diploma in Psychiatry, Edinburgh
1912	MRCP, Edinburgh
1912	Diploma in Psychological Medicine, London
1912	Gaskell Medal of the Medico — Psychological Association
1932	FRCP, London
1951	FRCP, Edinburgh
1955	FRCSC
1966	FRCS, Edinburgh

Positions Held
1908-9	House Officer, Edinburgh Royal Infirmary
1909-12	Assistant Medical Officer, Derby Borough Asylum
1912-13	Pathologist, Winwick Hospital, Warrington
1913-14	Pathologist, Wolverhampton Royal Infirmary
1914-15	Lieutenant, then Captain 3rd North Midland Field Ambulance attached to 3rd Field Ambulance Corps, 46th Division of Imperial Forces, Canadian Imperial Forces
1915-37	Professor of Pathology, University of Manitoba
1937-51	Professor of Pathology, University of Toronto
1951-54	Professor of Pathology, University of British Columbia
1956-60	Visiting Professor of Pathology, University of Alabama

Associations and Honours (Incomplete)
1934	President, American Association of Pathologists & Bacteriologists
1934	President, International Association of Medical Museums
1937	Fellow of the Royal Society of Canada

1937	LLD, University of Saskatchewan
1939-40	Chairman, Section of Pathology, Academy of Medicine, Toronto
1943-44	President, Ontario Association of Pathologists
1945-46	President, Toronto Academy of Medicine
1945	MD, University of Oslo
1947	Chairman, Committee on Cancer Control, Canadian Medical Association
1947	Director, National Cancer Institute of Canada
1950	President, National Cancer Institute of Canada
1956	LLD Queen's University, Kingston
1957	The William Wood Gerhard Gold Medal (Philadelphia Patholigical Society, for eminence in pathology)
1962	Gold-Headed Cane, American Association of Pathologists
1968	FNG Starr Award, Canadian Medical Association
1968	DSc, University of Manitoba
1968	Companion of the Order of Canada
1975	Honorary Fellow American College of Pathologists

Appendix 2

The Golden Chain: The Revisions of Boyd's Books

Year	Title	Edition
1916	*With a Field Ambulance at Ypres*	
1920	*Cerebrospinal Fluid*	
1925	*Surgical Pathology*	1st Ed.
1929	*Surgical Pathology*	2nd Ed.
1931	*Pathology of Internal Disease*	1st Ed.
1932	*Textbook of Pathology*	1st Ed.
1933	*Surgical Pathology*	3rd Ed.
1934	*Textbook of Pathology*	2nd Ed.
1935	*Pathology of Internal Disease*	2nd Ed.
1937	*Introduction to Medical Science*	1st Ed.
1938	*Surgical Pathology*	4th Ed.
1938	*Textbook of Pathology*	3rd Ed.
1939	Lectures in Pathology (Kansas)	
1940	*Pathology of Internal Disease*	3rd Ed.
1941	*Introduction to Medical Science*	2nd Ed.
1942	*Surgical Pathology*	5th Ed.
1943	*Textbook of Pathology*	4th Ed.
1944	*Pathology of Internal Disease*	4th Ed.
1945	*Introduction to Medical Science*	3rd Ed.
1947	*Textbook of Pathology*	5th Ed.
1947	*Surgical Pathology*	6th Ed.
1950	*Pathology of Internal Disease*	5th Ed.
1952	*Introduction to Medical Science*	4th Ed.
1953	*Textbook of Pathology*	6th Ed.
1955	*Surgical Pathology*	7th Ed.
1958	*Pathology for the Physician* formerly *Pathology of Internal Disease*	6th Ed.
1961	*Textbook of Pathology*	7th Ed.
1962	*Introduction to the Study of Disease* formerly *Introduction to Medical Science*	5th Ed.
1965	*Pathology for the Physician*	7th Ed.

1967	*Pathology for the Surgeon* formerly *Surgical Pathology*, (revised by W. Anderson)	8th Ed.
1970	*Textbook of Pathology*	8th Ed.
1971	*Introduction to the Study of Disease*	6th Ed.
1977	*Introduction to the Study of Disease* (with H. Sheldon)	7th Ed.
1980	*Introduction to the Study of Disease* (H. Sheldon)	8th Ed.
1984	*Introduction to the Study of Disease* (H. Sheldon)	9th Ed.
1988	*Introduction to the Study of Disease* (H. Sheldon)	10th Ed.
1990	*Textbook of Pathology* (revised by A.C. Ritchie)	9th Ed.

Appendix 3

Bibliography — 1907-1977 from *Toronto Academy of Medicine Bulletin* 52:112-115 1979, compiled by Dr. H.J. Barrie.

BOOKS:

With a Field Ambulance at Ypres, being letters written March 7—August 15, 1915, by William Boyd. New York: G.H. Doran Co., (c. 1916).

Physiology and Pathology of the Cerebrospinal Fluid. New York: Macmillan, 1920.

Surgical Pathology. Philadelphia: W.B. Saunders. 1st ed., 1925; 2nd ed., 1929; 3d ed., 1933; 4th ed., 1938; 5th ed., 1942; 6th ed., 1947; 7th ed., 1955; 8th ed. 1967 as *Pathology for the Surgeon.*

The Pathology of Internal Diseases. Philadelphia: Lea & Febiger. 1st ed., 1931; 2d ed., 1935; 3d ed., 1940; 4th ed., 1944; 5th ed., 1950; 6th ed., 1958 as: *Pathology for the Physician.* 7th ed. 1965.

Textbook of Pathology. Philadelphia: Lea & Febiger. 1st ed., 1932; 2d ed., 1934; 3d ed., 1938; 4th ed., 1943; 5th ed., 1947; 6th ed., 1953; 7th ed., 1961; 8th ed., 1970; 9th ed. rewritten by A.C. Ritchie 1990.

An Introduction to Medical Science. Philadelphia: Lea & Febiger. 1st ed., 1937; 2d ed., 1941; 3d ed., 1945; 4th ed., 1952; 5th ed., 1962 as *An Introduction to the Study of Disease*; 6th ed., 1971; 7th ed., 1977 with H. Sheldon.

Lectures in Pathology, by William Boyd. Delivered at the University of Kansas School of Medicine, Lawrence, Kansas City. Lawrence: University extension division, University of Kansas, 1939.

The Spontaneous Regression of Cancer. Springfield: Thomas, 1966.

ARTICLES

A case of general paralysis of the insane with extraordinary lymphocytosis in the cerebro-spinal fluid. *Br.M.J.* (1909) *1*: 1352-3.

A case of tumour of the pituitary body. *Lancet* (1910) *2*: 1129-31.

The cerebro-spinal fluid in health and disease. Gold Medal MD Thesis Edin. Univ., 1911.

A case of cerebral and crossed cerebellar hemiatrophy. *Rev. Neurol. Psych.* (1912) *10*: 318-25.

The cerebro-spinal fluid in certain mental conditions, *J. Ment. Sci.* (1912) *58*: 203-25; *Rev. Neurol. Psych.* (1912) *10*: 293 (abstract).

Leucytosis produced by the injection of normal saline solution. *J. Ment. Sci.* (1913) 59: 86.

_____, Hopwood, J.S. A case having a bearing on the localization of the auditory centre. *Lancet* (1913) 1: 1661.

On the occurrence of micrococci in the blood and cerebro-spinal fluid of two cases of mania. (with G.L. Brunton) *Br.M.J.* (1913) 2: 1212.

The clinical importance of the cerebro-spinal fluid. *Br. Med. J.* (1914) 1: 961.

Some sequelae of antityphoid inoculation. *Can. Med. Assoc. J.* (1915) 5: 398-404.

Certain peculiar crystals found in the cerebro-spinal fluid. *Lancet* (1915) 1: 993.

The clinical pathology of the cerebro-spinal fluid. *Can. Med. Assoc. J.* (1916) 6: 984-95.

A case bearing on the function of the pituitary body. *J.A.M.A.* (1917) 68: 111-3.

The present position of vaccine therapy. *Can. Med. Assoc. J.* (1918) 8: 706-17.

Acute adrenal insufficiency. *J. Lab. Clin. Med.* (1918) 4: 133-7.

Mackay, H., and _____. A contribution to the pathology of *mycosis fungoides*. *J. Cutan. Dis.* (1918) 36: 521-8.

Recent work on the chemistry of the blood and urine. *Can. Med. Assoc. J.* (1919) 9: 385-95.

Some uses of nonspecific protein therapy. *J. Lab. Clin. Med.* (1919) 5: 88-92.

The Winnipeg epidemic of encephalitis lethargica. *Can. Med. Assoc. J.* (1920) 10: 117-40.

Epidemic encephalitis; a study of seventy-five cases with sixteen autopsies. *Ann. Med.* (1920) 1: 195-221.

The sequelae of epidemic encephalitis. *Am. J. Med. Sci.* (1921) 162: 248-58.

Tissue resistance in malignant disease. *Surg. Gynecol. Obstet.* (1921) 32: 306-10.

The detection of *Lamblia (Giardia) intestinalis* by means of the duodenal tube. *Can. Med. Assoc. J.* (1921) 11: 658-60.

Gall-bladder problems. *Can. Med. Assoc. J.* (1922) 12: 689-93.

The preservation of amyloid specimens. *Bull.Int. Assoc. Med. Museums* (1922) 8: 77.

Paraffinoma, hydrocarbon fibromatosis. *Bull. Int. Assoc. Med. Museums* (1922) 8: 153.

The etiology of cancer. *Can. Med. Assoc. J.* (1922) 12: 421-2.

Studies in gall-bladder pathology. *Br. J. Surg.* (1922-3) 10: 337-56.

Epidemic encephalitis; the second Winnipeg outbreak. *Q.J. Med.* (1925) 18: 153-73.

Lansdowne, L.P. and _____. Congenital dilatation of the ureters. *Can. Med. Assoc. J.* (1925) 15: 361-6.

Diffuse tumors of the meninges. *Am. J. Pathol.* (1925) *1*: 583-93.

Three tumors arising from neuroblasts. *Arch. Surg.* (1926) *12*: 1031-48.

Williams, T.H. and _____. Spontaneous rupture of the oesophagus. *Surg. Gynecol. Obstet.* (1926) *42*: 57-60.

An address on nephrosis. *Can. Med. Assoc. J.* (1926) *16*: 349-52.

Acute myocardial syphilis. *Arch. Pathol. Lab. Med.* (1926) *2*: 340-2.

Lord Lister. *Lancet* (1927) *47*: 557-64.

Some points in the pathology of gall bladder. *Can. Med. Assoc. J.* (1927) *17*: 1015-18.

Notes on pathology of adenomatous goitre. *Trans. R. Soc. Can.* (1929) *23*: 289-91.

Students' conferences in teaching of pathology. *J. Tech. Methods & Bull. Int. Assoc. Med. Museums* (1929) *12*: 24-5.

Turvey, S.E.C. and _____. Three cases of endometriosis. *Can. Med. Assoc. J.* (1929) *21*: 304.

Immunological problems in septicaemia. *Br. Med. J.* (1930) *2*: 478.

Notes on the pathology of primary carcinoma of the lung. *Can. Med. Assoc. J.* (1930) *23*: 210-7.

The glioma group studied by ordinary histological methods. *Br. Med. J.* (1930) *2*: 720-2.

Hunter, C., McMillan, J.C., _____, and Cameron, A.J. Cortical adrenal tumour; clinical conference at Winnipeg General Hospital. *Can. Med. Assoc. J.* (1931), *25*: 188-93.

Endocarditis. *Lancet* (1931) *51*: 660-4.

The cells in the cerebrospinal fluid. In: Penfield, W.G., ed. *Cytology and cellular pathology of the nervous system.* 3 vols. New York: Hoeber, 1932.

Identity of adenoma of thyroid. *Trans. Assoc. Am. Physicians* (1932) *47*: 268-72.

Polycythemia, duodenal ulcer and coronary thrombosis. *Trans. Assoc. Am. Physicians* (1933) *48*: 209-11.

New form of museum catalogue. Int. Assoc. Med. Museums, *J. Tech. Methods & Bull. Int. Assoc. Med. Museums* (1934) *13*: 27-8.

Relationship of polycythemia to duodenal ulcer. *Am. J. Med. Sci.* (1934) *187*: 589-94.

Benign epithelial invasion. *Can. Med. Assoc. J.* (1934) *31*: 273-5.

Growth, innocent and malignant (Gordon Bell memorial lecture). *Can. Med. Assoc. J.* (1934) *31*: 124-130.

Idea of a clinical pathological museum. *J. Tech. Methods & Bull. Int. Assoc. Med. Museums* (1935) *14*: 10-8.

Growth, normal and abnormal. *J.A.M.A.* (1935) *105*: 1520-2.

Adamson, G.L., _____, and Cameron, A.J. Malignant disease and hypercalcaemia. *Can. Med. Assoc. J.* (1936) *35*: 308-10.

Museum as instrument in teaching of pathology. *J. Tech. Methods & Bull. Int. Assoc. Med. Museums* (1936) *16*: 1-4.

Group method in teaching of pathology. *J. Assoc. Am. Med. Colleges* (1937) *12*: 69-77.

James, E., and _____. Echinococcus alveolaris, with report of a case. *Can. Med. Assoc. J.* (1937) *36*: 354-6.

Growth — innocent and malignant. *Proc. R. Can. Inst.* (1938) *3*: (Ser. 3A), 63-6.

The general pathology of Cancer. In: *Handbook of Cancer*. Murray Printing Co., 1938, Chapter 1.

The early diagnosis of cancer. *Assoc. Med. Students Convention Book* (1938) *28-30*, 12.

Dr. Maude E. Abbott. *J. Tech. Methods & Bull. Int. Assoc. Med. Museums* (1938) *18*: 1-2.

Tumours and cysts of the neck. *Trans. West. Surg. Assoc., 1938* (1939) *48*: 172-82.

Some reasons for recent increase of bronchial carcinoma. (Thomas Dent Mutter Lecture) College of Physicians of Philadelphia, December 7th, 1938. *Trans. & Stud. Coll. of Phys. of Philadelphia* (1939) *6*: 317-2.

"Inflammation", from chapter on "Inflammation and Repair of Tissue". In: Christopher, Frederick, ed. *A textbook of surgery by American authors*. Philadelphia: Saunders, 1st ed., 1936; 2d ed., 1939; 3d ed., 1942; 4th ed., 1945; 5th ed., 1949, pp. 1-4.

The function of the museum in the medical school. *J.A.M.A.* (1941) *116*: 2545.

Sir Frederick Grant Banting 1891-1941. *Trans. Am. Assoc. Physicians* (1941) *56*: 9.

X-ray films in the pathological museum. *J. Tech. Methods* (1941) *21*: 18-20.

Functions of museum in medical school. *Proc. Ann. Cong. Med. Educ.* (1941) pp. 30-31.

Changing concepts of pyelonephritis. *Can. Med. Assoc. J.* (1942) *47*: 128-133.

Geographic pathology. *Can. Assoc. Med. Stud. Int. J.* (1943) *2*: 90-92.

Life blood. *Proc. R. Canad. Inst.* (Ser. 3A) (1942-3) *8*: 30-32.

Reasons for recent increase of bronchogenic carcinoma. *West. J. Surg.* (1944) *52*: 330-334. Also in *Proc. Calif. Acad. Med.* (1944) *8*: 9-13.

The education of a doctor — inaugural address of the President, *Acad. of Med. Bull.* (1945) *19*: 27-35.

Payne, J.F. and _____. Lucite in museum work. *J. Tech. Methods & Bull. Int. Assoc. Med. Museums* (1945) *25*: 79-80.

Coronary occlusion. *Bull. Acad. Med. Toronto* (1945) *18*: 173-176.

Recent advances in cancer research with special reference to cancer of the mouth. *J. Can. Dent. Assoc.* (1946) *12*: 539-42.

The problem of trauma and malignant disease in compensation work. *Bureau of Labor Standards, U.S. Dept. Labor, Bull. 94,* 1947.

Walker, G.R. and _____. Case of "double aorta" (Extensive healed dissecting aneurysm of the aorta). *Can. Med. Assoc. J.* (1948) *58*: 379-82.

Symposium on the cytologic diagnosis of cancer. Discussion of papers. *Am. J. Clin. Pathol.* (1949) *19*: 341-6.

The spread of tumours. In: Harris, R.I., ed. *Essays in surgery presented to Dr. W.E. Gallie.* Toronto: University of Toronto Press, 1950, pp. 358-75.

Pathology. *Univ. Toronto Med. J.* (1951) *29*: 89-93.

Pathology of ground substance mesenchyme. *Hawaii Med. J.* (1952) *11*: 353-357.

William Lipsett Robinson, 1885-1954. *J. Pathol. Bacteriol.* (1955) *70*: 257-8.

The spontaneous regression of cancer. *Can. Cancer Conf.* (1957) *2*: 354-60.

The Gordon Richards memorial lecture on the spontaneous regression of cancer: Part I; Introduction. *J. Can. Assoc. Radiol.* (1957) *8*: 45-9.

The Gordon Richards memorial lecture on the spontaneous regression of cancer: Part II; The meaning of spontaneous regression. *J. Can. Assoc. Radiol.* (1957) *8*: 63-7.

The medical society and the practice of medicine. *Can. Med. Assoc. J.* (1957) *76*: 439-42.

George Lyman Duff: in memoriam — first annual George Lyman Duff Memorial Lecture. *Can. Med. Assoc. J.* (1958) *78*: 962-3.

Spontaneous regression of cancer. *Med. Grad. (Toronto)* (1957-8) *4*: 6-11.

Spines I have known. *Med. Grad. (Toronto)* (1958-9) *5*: 7-14.

The development of cellular pathology. *Can. Med. Assoc. J.* (1963) *88*: 435-8.

Cause and effect: the fifth Alexander Gibson Memorial Lecture. *Can. Med. Assoc. J.* (1965) *92*: 868-74.

Pathology and disease. (editorial). *Univ. Toronto Med. J.* (1969) *66*: 182-3.

The medical museum. *J.Roy Coll. Surg. Edin.* (1972) *17*: 325-8.

Osler the candidate. *Can. Med. Assoc. J.* (1974) *111*: 393.

ADDENDA

On looking things up. *Univ. Manitoba Med. J.* (1931) *2*: 115-116.

On the dangers of scrappiness. *Univ. Manitoba Med. J.* (1937) *8*: 91-92.

Classification of epidermoid growths with some remarks on classification in general. *Can. J. Med. Technol.* (1941) *3*: 51-55.

Introduction 2: Classification and routes of spread of thoracic and intrathoracic tumors. In: G.T. Pack and I.M. Ariel. *Treatment of cancer and allied diseases.* 2d ed. Hoeber, 1960. v. 4, pp. 249-265.

Pathology: introductory lecture. *Univ. B.C. Med. J.* (1962) *1*: 5-9.

Index

American Association of Pathologists, 106
American Cancer Society meeting, 157
American Society of Physicians, 106
anti-Jewish sentiment, 90, 103
asylum physician, 53
Aszkanazy, Clarisse (Lore), 158
autopsies, 55, 56, 57, 104

Banting Institute, 133, 135
Barrie, John, 129, 172
Bell, Gordon, 78
Bell, Lennox, 166
Best, C.H., 134
books, 115 et sqq.
Boyd and his mother, 58
Boyd, Dugald Cameron, 13, 14, 19
Boyd, Elizabeth, 15
Boyd, gardener, 148, 166
Boyd, on medical education, 145
Boyd, organizer, 142
Boyd plagiarized, 129
Boyd's attitude to teaching, 106
Boyd's attitude to role of professional women, 158
Boyd's family, 25, 26
Boyd's first autopsy report, 56
Bramwell, Byron, 44
Butcher, Eliza Marion, 16

Cairo, 91
Cameron, A.T., 90
Canadian Cancer Society, The, 143
cerebrospinal fluid, 55, 116
childhood, 21
Chown, Henry H., 78, 93
climbing, 32, 33, 34, 35, 36, 87, 97, 98, 143
Commonplace Book, 47, 48
cost of living, 37
Croom, Halliday, 39

dancing, 38, 86
debating, 37
Department of Pathology, University of British Columbia, 155
Depression, The, 101
Derby, 47, 52

Edinburgh, 27
Edinburgh, Royal College of Surgeons, 162
Edinburgh Royal Infirmary, 30, 46
Elephant Man, 158
encephalitis lethargica, 89, 122
Enid, 81, 82, 83
epidemics, 74, 75, 90, 102
evangelical revivals, 19

field ambulance, 65
Flanders, 68, 75
Flexner commission, 76
Free Church of Scotland, 19

gallbladder, 118
Gallie, E.W., 134
gas attack, 68, 69
Gibson, Alexander, 29, 31, 72, 76
Gold-Headed Cane, 165
Graduation, 45
Grant, J.C.B., 31, 80, 86, 134
Greenfield, W.S., 29
Guy's Hospital, 109

Ham, A.W., 134

influenza, Spanish, 75
International Association of Medical Museums, 106

Jubilee, 103

Klotz, Oskar, 134

Lay Sermon, A., 163
Lea & Febiger, 97
Lederman, John, 87
Linell, Eric, 136

Machray embezzlement, 102
Manchester for radiotherapy, 151
Manitoba Medical College, 76, 103
Marrian, G.F., 134
Mayo, William J., 120
McEachern, John, 91
McManus, J.F.A., 160

MD thesis, 55
medical student, 27 et sqq.
Medovy, Harry, 96
Meltzer, S., 91
Michener, Rt. Hon. Roland, 171
Museum, Toronto, 137, 141, 152, 159
Museum, Vancouver, 159
Museum, Winnipeg, 90, 104, 105, 110
music, classical, 97

Nicholson, Daniel, 82, 87

old age, 170
Order of Canada, Companion of, 171
Organization Man, 142

Papers, 115
Pathologist, practising, 103
Pathology Building, new, 79
petitions, 108
Pierce, S.J.S., 78, 79
Portsoy, 13, 16, 17, 18, 19, 20
Postgraduate Medical School, London, 109
poverty in Winnipeg European immigrants, 74
Professor of Pathology, 77
Prowse, Dean, 82
public speaking, 37

Queen's University, Kingston, 128

retirement, 159
revising the books, 144
Robinson, William, 136

Saunders and Co., 97
Scrappiness, On the Dangers of, 111
siblings, 23
spontaneous regression of cancer, 124
Stanford University, 109
Stoloff, Cleone, 168

Toronto, 131
Toronto Academy of Medicine, 152
tumour, parotid, 150

University of Aberdeen, 109
University of Alabama, 159
University of British Columbia, 153 et sqq.
University of Toronto, 131 et sqq.

Vancouver General Hospital, 154

wedding, 86
Wiglesworth, F.W., 103
Winnipeg, 72 et sqq.
Winnipeg general strike, 75
Winwick Hospital, 60
Wolverhampton Royal Infirmary, 61
Words, 125, 174
World War II, 99, 140

Ypres, 64 et sqq., 115